From witch doctor to atomic scientist—here is a vivid history of the men and women who pioneered in the medical discoveries that have advanced the science and art of healing.

Jenner, Pavlov, Curie, Pasteur, Freud—this is their story. But it is also the story of the soldier who knew how to treat gout, the Bavarian physics professor who discovered X rays, the German bacteriologist who initiated the era of sulfa drugs, the Ohio convicts who volunteered for cancer research—all of the people who have contributed their knowledge, their skill, and their lives to the fight against disease.

The New York Times wrote, "Calder has demonstrated again that a good journalist who specializes in the popularization of science can enliven a difficult subject."

MEDICINE AND MAN

THE STORY OF THE ART AND SCIENCE OF HEALING

RITCHIE CALDER

 A SIGNET SCIENCE LIBRARY BOOK

Published by THE NEW AMERICAN LIBRARY

*SIGNET SCIENCE LIBRARY BOOKS are published by
The New American Library of World Literature, Inc.
501 Madison Avenue, New York 22, New York*

PRINTED IN THE UNITED STATES OF AMERICA

Contents

Part One

EYE OF NEWT
AND TOE OF FROG

> Medicine . . . learned from a monk how
> to use antimony, from a Jesuit how to
> cure agues, from a friar how to cut for
> stone, from a soldier how to treat gout,
> from a sailor how to keep off scurvy,
> from a postmaster how to sound the
> Eustachian tube, from a dairy-maid how
> to prevent smallpox, and from an old
> market woman how to catch the itch-
> insect. It borrowed acupuncture and the
> moxa from the Japanese heathen, and
> was taught the use of lobelia by the
> American savage.
>
> —OLIVER WENDELL HOLMES
> *Medical Essays*, Boston, 1883

1. THE AULD WITCH

The Auld Witch was our great-grandmother. None of
my generation ever saw her but she was as real to us as
though she sat at our family fireside. She has haunted
me in the most unlikely places—the middle of the Sahara, in the snow deserts of the Arctic, in the jungles of
the Equator, and in meetings of learned societies or when
I am just sitting in an armchair turning over the pages of
medical literature.

Then I find myself treading once again a long forgotten road in the Scottish hills—over the brow of Balma-
shanner, that Everest of infancy; along the lip of the slate
quarry, that Grand Canyon of boyish daring; past the
Cauldhame Woods, with a bit of a spurt because the
gypsies camped there; down the brae to the spinney; and
then, left, up the steep, breathless road to the whitewashed
cottar homes of Craichie.

There recollection pauses at a low-roofed house, with a
window full of exciting things—Cupid's Whispers, brandy

balls, imperial mints, hundreds-and-thousands, mottled soap, fire-lighters, and great coils of tobacco, like tarry rope. The bell tinkles as the door opens again on to warm smells which are the incense of memory.

"Aye, Lizzie!," my mother would say with that Scottish reticence which substitutes for an embrace.

"Aye, cousin!," would be the reply. "Bring the bairn ben the hoose."

And we would go through the shop into the parlor, with its box bed discreetly closed, its glinting brasses and china dogs, and the kettle (pretending we had been expected) steaming on the hob. The peat reek would catch my throat and Cousin Aggie would say: "That's a bad cough the wee laddie has, but we'll soon mend that."

And she would go off into the shop and there would be clinking of unseen jars and the deceptive promise of a handful of sweets or maybe even a bar of chocolate. Pshah! Licorice! and not even the sweet black kind like cobbler's wax but a fagot of little twigs.

"Chew that, laddie. 'Guid for the tubes and guid for the kidneys'—that's what the Auld Witch aye said aboot licoreesh root."

The Auld Witch! All her grandchildren who had known her called her that, including the one who became a dean of theology, and the other who became a Salvation Army commissioner.

"She looked like one," my reverend uncle once told me as we paced the lawns of McGill. "She sat huddled in the ingleneuk, muttering to herself and frightening me with those black eyes that glared under a lace cap."

Those black eyes still glare out of a family album of blue-eyed Scots. They are the eyes of a gypsy—as indeed she was, a real Romany. In a hungry winter her tribe, wandering through the hills, had abandoned her in her swaddling clothes on the doorstep of a humble cottage. In that kindly Scots family, she grew up and married one of the sons and became our great-grandmother. How she acquired the knowledge and the lore which gained her the reputation of a "witch" nobody knows. A romantic relative of mine, attributing to heredity characteristics more than modern science would do, and accepting the gypsies as being indeed Egyptians, once stretched her genealogy back to the dynasty of Neferirika-ra (2730 B.C.), to the first woman doctor in history—the Chief Physician of the

Pharaoh! It is much more likely that her gypsy blood and appearance made her "kenspeckle" (conspicuous) in that sober, God-fearing community; that she was consulted as a "spey-wife" and was shrewd enough to collect the country lore to support her reputation. And courageous enough!

It needed courage—for one of the relics preserved in my home town is the "Witches Bridle." This is a hinged ring, just big enough to go round the head. In front there is a spur, and behind, a chain. The spur held the tongue and acted as a gag and the chain was fastened to the stake at which the witches were burned, the "bridle" stifling their cries. And there was that spot which we children would never pass on a dark night—the "Witches' Howe." The last burning was in 1682 but the relics remained on public display as a warning to anyone rash enough to practice witchcraft.

Of course, in spite of her impression on her grandchildren and the morbid fascination the idea had for us great-grandchildren, she was not really a witch. She was the Wise Woman of her village. She was the best doctor they had. Perhaps she was not above spicing her simples with a bit of the supernatural—like collecting the herbs on the night of the full moon or muttering a few incantations to impress her patients with the virtues of her remedies—but she was, above all, the repository of the *materia medica* of the countryside. She kept no written record of her prescriptions (because she could neither read nor write) but many of them survived in the recollection of her grandchildren.

As the years have passed, that second-hand awe which I had for the Auld Witch has been replaced by a respect which grows with every new advance in medical science, because modern research is confirming so much of what she and the other Wise Women practiced as a lore.

Once, in the middle of the Sahara, I took a swig of warm, sweet-tasting water from a goatskin gourd. The taste was strangely familiar; it reminded me of those twigs in that little Scottish cottage; it was licorice. Yes, said my guide, it was a Berber practice. They added licorice because they said it made you pass less water, sweat less, and need less salt. That incident, in turn, was recalled, like the Auld Witch, by a learned article which I read in the *Lancet* with the forbidding title "Synergistic Action of

Liquorice, and Cortisone in Addison's and Simmonds's Disease," by J. G. G. Borst *et al*. It was discussing the property which licorice has, in common with the modern drug cortisone, of so acting on the kidneys that sodium chloride and water are retained and dehydration (as in Addison's disease) is reduced. The article did not discuss the other attributes of licorice, which modern medical textbooks call "demulcent and antibechic" and which my great-grandmother called "guid for the tubes" and therefore for a cough; nor the laxative effect which those licorice twigs used to produce in me on my four-mile tramp home.

The Auld Witch obviously knew the virtues of many things before they were given fancy formulae or labeled as proprietary medicines. She is known to have prescribed dandelion tea as a belly-balm and if you are suffering from "hepatic congestion" or "acid atonic dyspepsia" your present-day physician might prescribe *succus taraxici* if he knew his *materia medica* as well as my great-grandmother did when she brewed her dandelions. She administered fennel and rue for women's complaints, and, without ever having heard of Dr. Withering and his discovery of digitalis, she prepared foxglove infusions as a heart tonic and a treatment for dropsy. She forced fish oils down her children's throats long before the discovery of Vitamin A and Vitamin D, and treated burns with cold tea leaves a century before tannic-acid treatment for burns became fashionable. When penicillin became known, one of her grandchildren recalled that the Auld Witch had put molds on whitlows. I would give a lot to know whether she got the mold from the hyssop, because I could then stake the family claim to have discovered *penicillium notatum* and its antibiotic properties a century before Sir Alexander Fleming.

2. THE MEDICINE MAN

What a pity the Auld Witch never met her great American contemporary Oliver Wendell Holmes (*The Autocrat of the Breakfast-Table*)! While his predecessor at Harvard, Cotton Mather, would have had her burned at the stake, Holmes, a century ago, would have respected her as a fellow-physician.

Among the pompous practitioners of the nineteenth century, Holmes, at least, recognized that the top hat and frock coat of the doctor were as much the garb of the Medicine Man as the buffalo horns and skin of the Pawnee witch doctor. He would have seen in her simples the *materia medica* of his own craft. He would have recognized in her muttered "spells," as in the rituals of the primitive medicine man, the equivalent of his colleague's "bedside manner"—the legitimate psychological tricks by which doctors throughout the ages have established their authority over their patients and a belief in the efficacy of their drugs. The credulity of patients is, as any honest doctor would admit, an important part of the treatment.

Holmes, as professor of anatomy at Harvard from 1847 to 1882, inherited and acquired a great deal of knowledge of the structure of the human body, but he had few illusions about the limitations of medicine in treating ailments of that body. As he wrote in 1860: "Throw out opium, which the Creator himself seems to prescribe, for we often see the scarlet poppy growing in the cornfields, as if it were foreseen that wherever there is hunger to be fed there must also be pain to be soothed; throw out a few specifics which our doctor's art did not discover; throw out wine, which is a food, and the vapors which produce the miracle of anesthesia—and I firmly believe that if the whole *materia medica,* as now used, could be sunk to the bottom of the sea, it would be all the better for mankind—and all the worse for the fishes."

Medicine, in his time, was certainly not a science but rather a scrapbook of information and most of what was valuable had been discovered by people who were not primarily doctors. As he wrote: "Medicine appropriates everything from every source that can be the slightest use to anybody who is ailing in any way, or likely to be ailing from any cause. It learned from a monk how to use antimony, from a Jesuit how to cure agues, from a friar how to cut for stone, from a soldier how to treat gout, from a sailor how to keep off scurvy, from a postmaster how to sound the Eustachian tube, from a dairy-maid how to prevent smallpox, and from an old market woman how to catch the itch-insect. It borrowed acupuncture and the moxa from the Japanese heathen, and was taught the use of lobelia by the American savage."

3. THE MONK

Even that list is partly mythical. The "monk" was "Basil Valentine," who was supposed to have lived in the fifteenth century. This was more likely the pseudonym of an alchemist, Johann Thölde, who wrote in the early part of the seventeenth century. The origin of the name *antimony,* as given in his book *The Triumphant Chariot of Antimony,* published in 1604, was that "Valentine" had observed that some pigs which had eaten food containing antimony became very fat. He decided to try the effects on some monks who had become emaciated through fasting. They died. So with grisly humor he called it "antimoine," which means "anti-monk," or "monk's-bane."

As a matter of fact *antimony,* under the name *stibium,* had been known to Paracelsus (of whom we will hear much more). This was one of the metallic drugs (as distinct from herbal drugs) which he employed and which entitle him to be called the forerunner of modern chemotherapy.

It was, however, the bogus monk and the seventeenth-century "discovery" of his alleged fifteenth-century writings which started the cult of antimony, which persisted for centuries. As "tartar emetic" it was prescribed at the start of fevers, and its legendary effect on the monks probably was its actual effect on a very large number of patients—They died! Molière, convinced that the doctors had killed his only son with antimony, carried his grudge against the medical profession into five of his comedies, which satirized the doctor's pretensions and their ignorance. In Le Sage's *Gil Blas* there is a reference to "fellows in this town calling themselves physicians, who drag their degraded persons at the *Currus Triumphalis Antimonii,* or Cart's Tail of Antimony."

Was antimony a remedy or simply a poison? The controversy raged throughout the seventeenth century. Antimony, however, prevailed by royal patronage. Louis XIV became ill with typhoid fever and was given a dose of antimony. He recovered—therefore antimony must be a sovereign cure. This sort of reasoning was typical of the prescientific era in medicine. A person was ill; he was given something; he recovered; therefore "the something" was the cure for the complaint and would cure others in

14

the same way. The possibility that Louis XIV or whoever it was was already "on the mend" and would have recovered without the treatment was never considered. What we now call "controls" never occurred to doctors. In clinical tests today (apart from test-tube and animal experiments to avoid human risks) a new drug is administered to one group of patients and an inert substance to another group so that its efficacy can be studied not only in the patients who receive it but, by its absence, in the patients who don't. Without such a scientific method, doctors were no better than augurs reading signs and portents from individual cases, and if the case was "The Sun King"—Louis XIV—the "evidence" was assumed to be as absolute as the monarch.

Another French monarch, the Emperor Napoleon I, had no such faith in antimony. In exile on St. Helena, he suffered from a stomach complaint, either cancer or a gastric ulcer, and his medical attendant treated him with tartar emetic (antimony). Napoleon was convinced that he was being poisoned and on one occasion made his attendant drink the medicine. Montholan thus became violently ill. The ex-Emperor's worst suspicions were confirmed and he refused to have anything more to do with his physician. If, however, poison was being administered it was only because antimony was hallowed by medical sanction.

4. THE JESUIT

And now "the Jesuit who taught the doctors how to cure agues": *Quinine* came into European medical practice as "Jesuit's Bark"—(and because of its name, the Protestant Oliver Cromwell preferred the ague to the treatment). Like so much in medicine, quinine is wrapped up in legends. One thing which is certain is that it was derived from the Peruvian Indians. A plausible explanation of its name is that a Jesuit Father, working among the Indians in the high Andes was attacked by feverish ague of which he would have died if the local medicine man of the Incas had not brewed him a bark tea. He recovered and (so the story goes), having failed to persuade the medicine man to part with the secret of the remedy, he employed his convalescence in keeping observation, discovered how the bark was obtained, helped himself to some of it and smuggled it back to Lima.

A romantic embellishment of the legend is the story of the beautiful Countess of Cinchona, the wife of the Royal Governor of Peru. She was sick, and dying, of the fever. Neither the treatments of the court doctors nor the prayers of the priests could avail. Then at the critical moment an Indian arrived breathless from the mountains with slivers of tree bark. In spite of the protests of his doctors and of his priests at the use of heathen ritual, the Viceroy, in desperation, agreed to try this remedy. The beautiful Countess recovered.

The only thing wrong with this touching account is that it never happened. Spoilsport historians have proved that the Countess of Cinchona never went to Peru and never had malaria and consequently never needed "fever-bark," but the legend has probably been perpetuated forever because Linnaeus, the great Swedish botanist, accepted it and classified the fever-bark tree as "cinchona," after her, and "quinine" is a corruption of that.

Quinine, tincture of cinchona, was introduced into Europe in 1632. Its impact was sensational. It has been said: "Cinchona did for medicine what gunpowder had done for war." It upset all the existing systems of medicine as cannon had upset the feudal system.

It was a gift to the quacks. In England, Robert Talbot, who had been an apothecary's apprentice and who "qualified" as a doctor merely by putting up his shingle, invented a marvelous remedy (it was just rose leaves, lemon juice, water and quinine) which relieved intermittent fevers in a few days while the then conventional treatments took months. The plausible quack gained access to Charles II, cured him of a fever, and was knighted. Then the Dauphin and Dauphine of France were sick and dying of the fever when Talbot arrived at Versailles and was received in audience by Louis XIV, that "sucker" for quacks. He staked his head that he would cure the patients within four days. He did and was made a Chevalier, and handsomely rewarded by the king.

Like all new discoveries (even today) quinine was, of course, abused. It was regarded as a cure-all, and prescribed for diseases for which it had no value, and was given in excess, with ill effects. It took its proper place in medical practice through that wise clinician Thomas Sydenham (1624-1689). It remained a specific treatment for malaria, the shaking fever, improved a generation ago when the chemist made its application more effective by extracting its special virtues, and now, its method of action (on the parasite of malaria) having been learned, it has been replaced by new synthetic drugs.

5. THE SOLDIER

Thomas Sydenham was that "soldier who taught doctors how to treat gout" referred to by Oliver Wendell Holmes. He was a trooper in Cromwell's army during the British Civil War. Historians call him "a trooper turned physician."

As a physician, he remains an exemplar for all his kind. His ideas about medicine were as simple as his own nature. He had no use for scientific theories, or the hocuspocus which masqueraded as scientific theories in those days. His was the Hippocratic method, by-passing all the scholasticism and obscurantism of the Middle Ages back to the "Father of Medicine," Hippocrates (460-370 B.C.), who gave Greek medicine its scientific spirit and the medical profession, for all time, its ethical ideals.

Like Hippocrates, Sydenham "returned to the bedside." His textbook was his patient and each patient was a new volume to be studied with care. He relied, as good doctors must, on his powers of observation and his fund of related experience. He forsook the magic and mythology of medicine and insisted that disease was a natural process and not a supernatural visitation. He maintained that every disease belonged to a certain definite species, which could be described and classified as a botanist does plants.

When one considers the time in which he lived, his insight was remarkable. His studies of the geography and meteorology of epidemic diseases and how they recurred periodically were the basis of modern epidemiology. His clinical notes, first-hand accounts of diseases, were those of a superb observer. He described malaria, scarlet fever, measles, pneumonia, dysentery, chorea and hysteria.

His treatise on gout (1683) is regarded as his masterwork—and was obviously what impressed Holmes. That treatise was written with feeling.

"The physician must bear in mind," wrote Sydenham,

"that he is subject to the same laws of mortality and disease as others and so he will care for the sick with more tenderness if he remembers that he is himself their fellow-sufferer." That was the voice of experience. Sydenham himself suffered from gout for over thirty years and, in the end, he was forced out of practice by arthritis.

Gout, then as now, was an excruciatingly painful disease, which, as Sydenham pointed out, "afflicted the rich more frequently than the poor and rarely attacked fools." Treatments were as ruthless as the pains themselves.

Both *moxa* and *acupuncture,* which Holmes includes in his catalogue of borrowed medical practice, were employed as drastic remedies for gout. Moxa, which he attributes to the Japanese, had probably a much more remote origin. Sydenham thought that he recognized it as a treatment used by Hippocrates. The Egyptians had something like it and so did the Chinese, from whom the Japanese may have learned it. Acupuncture was (and still is) an accepted Chinese practice. Both seem pretty drastic remedies. Moxa consists of cones of combustible material applied, like candles on a birthday cake, to the affected part and lit. "Acupuncture" means sticking needles into the body. They are counterirritants (pain to counteract pain) although there may be more to acupuncture than that. Throughout the centuries, the Chinese have made a medical art of it. Students—eighteen hundred years ago—were taught acupuncture from a bronze image of the body with needle holes for each of the prescribed treatment points. This was something very different from the black magic which makes waxen images of an enemy into which pins are stuck to induce his destruction. In the Chinese scripts on acupuncture there is an immense amount of sound anatomy and, among the modern Chinese, acupuncture is being examined as a serious science. If needling has survived as a treatment for so long—perhaps accompanied by a good deal of incidental nonsense and abuses—there may be some entirely rational explanation of its effects from which modern science might profit. It is also of note that moxa was used, after the bombing of Hiroshima and Nagasaki, to treat atomic wounds.

But in Sydenham's day, moxa and acupuncture for gout was no more than lighting fires or sticking nails into the painful part. Sometimes, too, gout victims would submit themselves to being parboiled in steam chambers as a "sweat treatment." They would suffer bloodletting and purging to dangerous, and often fatal, extremes. Sydenham, the wise physician, distrusted and rejected such excesses. For gouty patients, he recommended diet and rest, fresh air and horseback riding, and moderation in all things. One of his own remedies (for himself) was a "draught of small beer," which he took before dinner, after dinner and before going to bed. But, while he recognized that the gross drinking habits of the wealthy was probably one of the causes of their gout, he coined the phrase which is still medically valid. "If you drink wine, you have the gout. If you do not drink wine, the gout has you."

Thomas Sydenham preached temperance not only in winebibbing but in medical prescribing. The pharmacopoeia to which, in his day, his contemporaries turned for their prescriptions reads like a collection of sewage. At a time which we regard as the dawning of modern science, with the founding of the Royal Society and the like, we find the doctors prescribing *live worms*; lozenges of dried *vipers; foxes' lungs* (for asthma); *powdered gems; oil of bricks; oil of ants; oil of wolves; butter made in May; bile, viscera, claws, teeth, hoofs, sexual organs, excreta of animals, human urine, human placenta; raw silk, spiders' webs, sponge; human perspiration; saliva from a fasting man; cast-off snake's skins; swallows' nests; wood lice; moss* from the skull of a victim of violent death or *part of the skull* of an executed criminal.

We find the Royal Society being asked to report on the efficacy of unicorn horn as an antidote to poison, and one of its distinguished fellows, Governor John Winthrop of Connecticut, accepting unicorn horn for use in his medical practice. We find *bezoar stone* still in use, again as an antidote to poison. This was a legacy of the Arabs. The stones were reputed to be the petrified tears of a stricken stag, but were in fact concretions formed in the intestines of animals—often gallstones.

Sydenham could not entirely escape the claptrap of his times, but he reverted to vegetable simples, accepted the new properties of quinine, recognized the value of iron tonic in anemia, and treated syphilis with mercury.

His reputation as a practitioner was so great that Boerhaave of Leyden, the finest medical teacher in Europe, would bare his head at the very mention of his name. His attitude towards his craft (for it still was not a science), and to his contemporaries, is summed up in the account of his meeting with Hans Sloane. Sloane, about to become one of the fashionable and wealthy physicians and founder of the British Museum, went to Sydenham's house, in Pall Mall, London, with a letter of introduction which described him as "a ripe scholar, a good botanist and a skillful anatomist."

Sydenham threw the letter aside in contempt and exclaimed "This won't do—Anatomy! Botany! Nonsense! Sir, I know an old woman in Covent Garden who understands botany better. As for anatomy, my butcher can dissect a joint full as well. No, young man, all this is stuff; you must go to the bedside, for it is there alone that you can learn disease."

In spite of this unpromising reception, Sloane became a resident pupil in Sydenham's house, and went on to become physician to the King, President of the Royal Society (in succession to Sir Isaac Newton), Academician of France, and President of the Royal College of Physicians.

6. *ROBINSON CRUSOE*

Another resident pupil of Sydenham's had a less honorific but much more colorful career—as a buccaneer and as the man who rescued "Robinson Crusoe."

This was Thomas Dover (1662-1742) who, when he left Sydenham's kindly home and enlightened teaching, settled in the port of Bristol as a doctor. There he saw an opportunity of getting rich more quickly than by bleeding and purging the merchant princes. To say that he became a pirate is untrue—but only barely so. He engaged in piracy for which he could not be hanged at Execution Dock, because he sailed under the King's license, with Woodes Rogers, to pillage ships as a privateer. At least one bishop and several church dignitaries helped to finance the buccaneering enterprise and shared the rich spoils with Dover and his shipmates.

The *Duke* and *Duchess,* the two frigates engaged for the voyage, set sail on August 1, 1708, with Dr. Dover as Second Captain to Woodes Rogers on a voyage which was to last three years. By looting Spanish traders, attacking French men-of-war, pillaging cities along the west coast of South America, and adventuring along the coasts of California, the privateers acquired a fortune in "prizes," of £170,000 after meeting all expenses. Licensed piracy was a profitable undertaking.

On January 21, 1709, the ships were abreast the island of Juan Fernández. Both the ships and the crews were in pretty poor shape through lack of fresh meat and the spread of scurvy. Woodes Rogers was chary about landing on this unpredictable island; there might be French or Spaniards waiting in ambush there. Dover, forgetting that he was only Second Captain and remembering, as a doctor, the plight of the crew, insisted on taking the pinnace and going ashore to reconnoiter. He was so impatient that he set out when darkness was about to fall, and, as the pinnace neared the shore, a light appeared on the island. This so startled the boat crew that they insisted on turning back to their armed ships.

Next morning the frigates crept cautiously round the island but could see no signs of any inhabitants or any explanation of the fire of the previous night. So Dover and his landing party ventured ashore. They found the explanation of the lights—a strange figure clad in goatskins, who became familiar to generations of children as "Robinson Crusoe."

He was actually Alexander Selkirk, of Largo, Fifeshire, Scotland, who claimed to have been Master of the ship *Cinque Ports*. His story was disconnected and his speech uncertain, because he had forgotten how to communicate with his fellow humans. He insisted, however, that four years and four months previously, he had been marooned by his captain after a quarrel. He had been put ashore with some ship's clothes and bedding, and a "firelock, some powder, bullets and tobacco, a hatchet, a knife, a kettle, a Bible, and some mathematical instruments and books." He had built himself two huts with pimento trees, covered them with grass and lined them with the skins of goats, which at first he shot with his gun, but later caught by chasing them on foot. At first he suffered extreme hunger because loneliness and lack of bread and salt made food unappetizing. He managed to eat giant crawfish but other sea food, without salt was at first unpalatable. His only companions were the goats and cats and rats. The cats and rats had escaped from ships which, at some time, had watered there, and they had bred in large numbers—like the goats which had been similarly marooned. To entertain himself, he danced with his cats. When his clothes wore out, he made himself coverings with goatskins sewn together with skin thongs, using a nail for a needle.

That story, duly embellished, but true in origins, became the famous novel of Daniel Defoe, the theme of pantomimes and the perennial adventure story of all children. But it did not sound plausible to Woodes Rogers and Dover, until, by a circumstance which so often makes fact stranger than fiction, it was fully confirmed by Dampier, one of the officers of the expedition. He revealed that he had been on the sister ship of the *Cinque Ports,* had known about the marooning but had never dared disclose it, and identified the Goat Man as, indeed, Alexander Selkirk, an excellent and ill-done-by seaman. On that recommendation, Woodes Rogers made the castaway mate of the *Duke.* Selkirk shared in the spoils but later regretted that he had ever forsaken his solitude.

Dover intrudes upon this book on medicine, however, not as the buccanneer-doctor, nor as the discoverer of "Robinson Crusoe" but because he is a link not only with the soldier from whom medicine learned to treat gout (Sydenham) but with another medical discovery which Oliver Wendell Holmes ought to have included in his list.

In most modern pharmacopoeias or medical formularies or dictionaries, you will still find "Dover's powder." The name has perpetuated this same Thomas Dover who first compounded "ipec. et. op." (ten per cent each of ipecacuanha and opium, with eighty per cent of sulfate of potassium). It is to be found (among the spiders' webs, the virgin's milk, the wood lice and the moss from human skulls) in Hans Sloane's London Pharmacopoeia of 1721, and is significant because it restored ipecacuanha to its rightful place in medical treatment.

Nobody knows how ipecacuanha reached Europe from Brazil. It is another drug which we owe to the South American Indians, who used it both as a poison and as a "sickmaker" or emetic. That is what the word originally meant—"roadside sickmaker." It was known to doctors in Paris in 1672, but its success was due to the Swiss quack Helvetius. Once again, the "experimental animal" was that same Dauphin who had been cured of the fever by Talbot's quinine administrations. Now he had dysentery. Helvetius, no doubt with serious misgivings, used ipecacuanha. Perhaps his success with his royal patient was due to his misgivings, for he used it in diffident quantities. Anyway, it worked, and once again the impressionable Louis XIV (antimony, quinine and now ipecacuanha) was duly grateful. He bought the "secret" remedy from Helvetius for 20,000 francs—a lot of money at that time. Its disclosure proved a poor public service because, once again, the doctors ran amok and administered "ipec." in lethal doses until Dover "tamed" it, limited its proportions, and used it to modify, in turn, the effects of opium.

Oliver Wendell Holmes might have included it both as a proper tribute to the Indian donors and as part of his other category—"the few specifics which our doctors' art did not discover" and which were in the physicians' black bags a century ago. But with this qualification—in 1820, François Magendie, of Bordeaux, had isolated "emetine" from ipecacuanha and had given the doctors that chemical essence of the drug which made it more effective in treating amoebic dysentery.

7. THE SAILOR

"From a sailor how to keep off scurvy"—now whom would the old "Autocrat" mean? Because there is a full quarter-deck of sailors who might deserve that credit. There was Cartier on his second voyage to Newfoundland in 1535. Scurvy broke out on his ship and one hundred of his one hundred and three men were desperately ill and in anguish. The Iroquois Indians of Quebec came to the rescue with "miraculous results." They provided an infusion of bark and leaves of the hemlock tree. Then Admiral Sir Richard Hawkins, in 1593, recorded that within his own personal experience 10,000 seamen had died of scurvy and, in his observations, recorded this significant statement: "That which I have seen most fruitful for this sickness is sower oranges and lemons."

The classic work was that of James Lind, a British naval surgeon, who became the chief physician of the Naval Hospital at Portsmouth. In 1753, he published a book showing how scurvy could be eliminated by supplying sailors with lemon juice. In this book, he quoted the case of a scurvy-stricken sailor in the Greenland ships of 1734 who was in such a bad way that his shipmates marooned him to die. He had almost lost the use of his limbs, but when he was put ashore he managed to crawl to a clump of grass on which he "grazed like a beast of the field." It acted like a charm. In a short time he was "perfectly recovered and upon his returning home it was found that it was the herb, scurvy grass."

Lind, by direct treatment at sea, proved the curative value of simple things like mustard cress, tamarinds, oranges and lemons (in fact, anything, as we know now, which contains the vitamin C of fresh fruit or herbs). He was, however, frustrated and remarked bitterly: "Some persons cannot be brought to believe that a disease so fatal and so dreadful can be cured or prevented by such easy means. They would have more faith in an elaborate composition dignified with the title of 'an antiscorbutic golden elixir' or the like." The "some persons" of his complaint were My Lords of the Admiralty, who ignored Lind's advice for forty years—and that despite the epic experience of Captain James Cook, on his expedition towards the South Pole and round the world. There was no scurvy on board the *Resolution* because he took Lind's advice and shipped fresh fruit. Captain Cook received the gold medal of the Royal Society and was made a Fellow, not for his adventurous voyages but for his scientific observation and his application of the simple remedy. But My Lords of the Admiralty did not read the proceedings of the Royal Society for 1776, any more than they had read the Lind reports. It was not until 1794, the year of Lind's death, that the first naval squadron was supplied with lemon juice for a twenty-three-week voyage and, despite the complete absence of scurvy on that voyage, it took another ten years for regulations enforcing consumption of daily rations of lemon juice, to be applied to the entire fleet. Then, and only then, did scurvy disappear from the British Navy and, after the lapse of another sixty years, the Board of Trade applied the same ordinances to all merchant ships.

That is why Americans call the British "limeys." The lemon was often called "lime" and this led to unfortunate confusions, because lime juice is inferior, in the prevention of scurvy, to lemon juice. But the nickname applied on the waterfronts to the British seamen, toping their "juice," has stuck.

8. THE POSTMASTER

"From a postmaster how to sound the Eustachian tube." In Holmes's quiz game, that is an easy one. The answer is Edme-Gilles Guyot, postmaster of Versailles, in 1724.

Guyot, in that year, was a very miserable *receveur des postes*. He was growing deaf. He kept hearing noises "in his head" and was afraid that he was going mad or was beset by devils. The doctors were no use to him. The honest ones told him that nothing was really known about the ear or about deafness and that anyone who pretended otherwise was a quack. The quacks pretended to treat him. The priests told him that deafness was a natural affliction and that he must accept it with pious resignation.

Guyot was not irreverent, but he was persistent. He by-passed the doctors and went to the source books. Treatment might be backward but anatomy was relatively well-advanced, and at length he discovered in the works of Eustachius (a contemporary of Vesalius of whom we shall hear more anon) his description (1563) of the tube, or canal, which runs from the throat to the middle ear. If one could breathe tobacco smoke, as the Court dandies did, from the mouth through the ears, there must be a through passage of some sort. He also noticed that he had a feeling of compression in his ears (a sensation which air travelers now experience when they are taking off or landing) and formed his own theory: If the Eustachian tube had any function it must be to carry air from the nose and throat to the middle ear and that air must, therefore, be necessary for good hearing. M. Guyot was also very conscious of his chronic catarrh, and decided that, somehow, the catarrh was blocking the Eustachian tube.

How to clear it? If hearing is affected by air pressure, as in flying, we know (nowadays) that the simple device is to hold the nostrils, close the mouth and force the air in the mouth up the tubes. But that was not the problem of the postmaster of Versailles. A man of resource, he devised a curved tube of tin which he could put into his mouth and insert in the opening of the Eustachian

canal. He padded it with leather so that it would not lacer-
ate or irritate his throat. This catheter he attached to a
reservoir with two pumps, operated by a crank. This
sounds grossly mechanical when we think of the rubber
bulb of a syringe which would serve the same function.
But he did manage to scour his Eustachian tube with this
device and he did recover his normal hearing. He washed
out of his head the devils of the priests and the ignorance
of the doctors.

The latter, at least, had the grace to be impressed and
the local postmaster was asked to read a paper and to
demonstrate his apparatus before the French Academy of
Sciences.

9. THE DAIRY-MAID

"From a dairy-maid, medicine learned how to prevent
smallpox"? Jenner, of course, and the discovery of vaccination. Or should it be Benjamin Jesty, the Dorset-
shire farmer?

It had long been the tradition of the English countryside that a milkmaid could catch a pustular eruption, like
a mild smallpox, from milking a cow infected with cowpox
and that, once she had that, she would be immune from
smallpox—that universal disease which killed or disfigured
rich and poor alike.

For the record, Benjamin Jesty, in 1774, took cowpox
matter from a pustule on the nipple of a cow and introduced it under the skin on the arms of his wife and two
of his sons. The sons had a mild reaction but that of Mrs.
Jesty was so severe that it did not encourage the country
folks to repeat the experiment. But the Jestys certainly
escaped smallpox.

Edward Jenner (1749-1823) hit upon this idea quite
independently. The son of a clergyman, he had been ap-
prenticed in medicine under the great John Hunter, who
esteemed him highly. But Jenner rejected the prospects of
a fashionable London practice and became a country doctor in his native county of Gloucestershire.

In May 1796, Jenner examined the hand of Sarah
Nelmes, a dairymaid near Berkeley, in Gloucestershire.
She had an eruption on her wrist and forefinger and at
the base of the thumb. Jenner had already made up his
mind that there was an affinity between cowpox and

mallpox and was convinced that the defenses of the body, once mobilized to resist and overcome the milder animal form, would repel the more virulent human version. With his conviction, he took some matter from the pustules of Sarah Nelmes and inserted it in the arm of a small boy, James Phipps. On the seventh day, James complained of a discomfort in the armpit, and an eruption appeared, scarred and healed, and left him none the worse.

This was satisfactory so far as it went but there was no proof that he was now immune from smallpox. On July 1, 1796, Jenner took the next drastic step. He transferred virulent infection from a person with smallpox to the boy Phipps. No disease followed, as, ordinarily, it would have been bound to do. And to make doubly sure, the boy was again inoculated a few months later without effect.

The doctor at least had dealt scientifically with a problem with which the yeoman farmer Jesty had adventurously experimented. It should be added that when, years later, the Jennerian Society invited Jesty and his son to London to acknowledge his kinship to the discovery, the son agreed to submit to the Phipps test. With faith in his father and in vaccination, he submitted to an inoculation of live smallpox and was found to be still immune—after an interval of years which the United States immigration officers would not nowadays accept on a vaccination certificate.

10. THE OLD MARKET WOMAN

"From an old market woman, medicine learned how to catch the itch-insect." Let it be quite clear that Oliver Wendell Holmes was referring not to flea-hunting or delousing, but to something which throughout the ages had discomforted the public and discomfited the doctors. Oh, yes, it was uncleanliness, but it was not simply that, nor was it due to fleas or lice. Itching and scratching had been the commonplace of rich and poor throughout the centuries. It was the reason for those elegant ivory forks which the Chinese had devised as back-scratchers and which, with the silks and scents and spices, had come to Europe as a fashionable accessory to be sported as nonchalantly as a lady's fan. It had been one of the reasons for the Roman baths, where to the hygiene of washing was added the hedonistic pleasure of luxurious scratching.

We know it now as "scabies," which is something one does not discuss in front of the neighbors. To call someone "scabrous" is to invite a sock in the jaw or a legal action. Not so among our forefathers, for "the itch" was a universal complaint to which all flesh was apparently heir.

In the early nineteenth century, the itch was a fashionable disease—a conversation-piece as our slipped disks or our friends' complexes are today—and courtiers would compare symptoms and itchiness with relish. Moreover it had given rise to a whole theory of disease—"the internal itch," or *gale répercutée,* which assumed that most of the diseases of the body were variations of the ever-present itch. Now, of course, we know, in these days of allergies and advanced dermatology, that itching skin can be traced to internal disorder; then the converse was believed.

The notion then current was all the more unpardonable because, away back in 1162, in the golden age of Arabian medicine of the Western Caliphate, Avenzoar, of Seville, had identified and described the itch-mite, and Wichmann, in 1786, had established the parasitic origin of scabies.

The itch-cult persisted, however, and one of its great exponents was "Jolly old Baron Alibert, with his broad-brimmed hat worn a little jauntily, calling out to the students in the courtyard of the Hospital St. Louis in Paris— 'Enfants de la méthode naturelle, êtes-vous tous ici?'" (to quote Oliver Wendell Holmes). And when the "children of the natural method" were all there—overflowing the courtyard where he had to hold his lectures because they were so popular—he would expound. He produced a "family tree" which made all skin-diseases kin. It was one of those confident, complacent concepts which characterized the dogmatic medicine of the early nineteenth century.

This complacency was, however, wrecked by one of Alibert's own students—a young Corsican named Renucci. He watched the Doctor-Baron build up a whole structure of theory on the basis of his total ignorance of how those pustules and scabs of the itch arose on the hands.

At last, inviting a Jovian thunderbolt, he challenged his professor. He knew, he said, what caused the itch because he had seen and learned from a market woman in a village square in Corsica. The Baron accepted the challenge good humoredly. A case of the itch was found—that was not difficult—and the student took a needle, pricked the blob, and speared a little red speck. He had extracted the itch-mite, just as the market woman had done.

To the credit of the bluff Baron Alibert, he afterwards used this demonstration to destroy the cult of the "internal itch" and to clear the way for systematic medicine based on experimental evidence instead of unsubstantial theories.

11. THE HEATHENS

What have we left of Holmes's catalogue? The "friar who cut for stone" has been overlooked. He was Frère Jacques de Baulot (1651-1719) a wandering friar who "went about cutting charitably for stone as the poor implored him." Acupuncture, we have dealt with. And moxa. That leaves lobelia, the use of which was "taught by the American savage." Lobelia was derived from the North American Indians who used the leaves and tops of a common weed as the Auld Witch, my great-grandmother, used her herbals. But lobelia, like so many beneficial plants, is treacherous in the wrong hands. In very large doses it can paralyze the heart's action, but in mild doses it relieves the spasms of asthma. Today, lobelia, the gift of the Indian, is used to discourage the habit of smoking—that other gift of the Indian.

There are a few other things which Holmes might have included—with a passing nod at the Auld Witch and her like. Notably, there was *digitalis* which Dr. William Withering, the good physician of Birmingham, got from a Shropshire wise woman. He watched her brewing foxglove tea and learned that the infusion was the local treatment for dropsy. Without knowing the distinction between cardiac dropsy (the accumulation of water in the body tissue owing to heart trouble) and renal dropsy (due to kidney failure), he started applying the virtues of the foxglove to heart cases and discovered its efficacy in certain types. Digitalis was one of the few specifics available to doctors a century ago. (A "specific" is a remedy which has a recognizable curative effect for a particular disease—treating the cause and not the symptoms.)

Holmes might also have included *mercury* for syphilis —going back to Paracelsus (1493-1541) who acquired so much of his knowledge and permanent contributions to medicine by collecting information from barbers, executioners, miners, bathkeepers, midwives, gypsies, mountebanks and fortunetellers. But, however Paracelsus acquired the knowledge of mercury, there is no doubt that preparations of it were in use in India in remote times.

A century ago, Oliver Wendell Holmes, Sr., looked in the doctor's black bag and found precious little there. In 1933, when his son, Mr. Justice Holmes, of the Supreme Court of the United States, died at the age of ninety-four, the doctors who attended him had very little more. Oh, yes, medical science had advanced; knowledge of the workings of the human body had increased; public health, nutrition, and the study of man's mind and behavior had made great strides; surgeons, with asepsis (which Oliver Wendell Holmes had advocated, in ignorance of germs and against the diatribes of his profession) and anesthetics (a word he invented), had adventured into the body. New words filled the medical textbooks—radiology, endocrinology, serology, psychology and -ology after -ology.

By 1933, the age of the specialist was upon us and that of the physician was in decline. As Lord Horder, the great clinician, said at the Medical Society of New York in 1936: "I regard this spread of specialization as being no less dangerous to the public than it would be for the passengers of a ship if the captain left the bridge and the chief engineer, or the chief steward, or the radio-operator, took his place."

Yet, by present-day standards, the general practitioner in the early 1930s was ill-equipped. A few years ago, I addressed the august Hunterian Society of London and, taking my life in my hands, dared to say: "Up to 1935, the physicians were merely witch doctors. They treated symptoms, not causes, of disease. They gave sedatives or stimulants, as the case might be. The doctors had about five specifics—quinine for malaria; ipecacuanha (or its derivative, emetine) for amoebic dysentery; and Paracelsus's mercury or Ehrlich's 'salvarsan' to attack the spirochaete of syphilis. Of those only salvarsan was recent. Most were of ancient origin. . . ."

In the early thirties, over 50 per cent of the drugs in

current use had been employed by Arab-speaking physicians in the Middle Ages, and two-thirds of those had been known to the later Greeks. The pharmacists of Main Street were dispensing drugs mentioned in the Egyptian papyri, including the familiars: aloes, caraway, coriander, dill, fennel, juniper, mint, myrrh and turpentine; and Ancient Egyptians had also bequeathed us salts of copper and of lead. The Assyrians had contributed, among many others, almond oil, aniseed, galbanum, and licorice; and Assyrian mineral remedies included alum and bitumen. The Indians, in their remote past, had given *cannabis indica* (hashish), cardamoms (for flatulence and spasms), senna pods, jimson weed (narcotic and antispasmodic) and nux vomica (containing strychnine and brucine). Dioscorides, a physician with the armies of Nero (in the first century A.D.), had collected 600 plants in his herbal, including opium and mandrake as narcotics. He had classified the plants according to the complaints for which they were serviceable and about a hundred of them are still in the *materia medica* of the profession.

12. JOYFULL NEWES

It is a quaint thought that America itself was a medical discovery. Yet, in a sense, it is true. Columbus was seeking a short cut to the spices of the East and "spices" were not then primarily the condiments and seasonings to which we apply the name today. Then, as now, men searched the ends of the earth for substances to assuage their ailments and temper their physical distresses. The bills of lading of the spice ships were more for the apothecaries than for the grocers—aloes, opium, benzoin, camphor, cubebs, musk (for hysteria), balsam resins, cinnamon and cloves. For such a trade, the Venetians fought the Turks and the Genoese, and became the wealthiest city on earth until, in 1498, Vasco da Gama rounded the Cape of Good Hope and opened the sea route to the East Indies. The center of the drug trade then became Lisbon and, with the rich inducements, not of Eldorado gold but of the drug trade, Columbus sought the westward route and opened up the American continents.

Because nutmegs are not as glamorous as gold, history which has romanticized the Spanish Main has tended to forget that one of the great naval epochs was the six-teenth-century domination by the Dutch of the spice routes and the drug marts, with bitter battles until, as Motley has said, "The world's destiny seemed almost to have become dependent upon the growth of a particular gillyflower." Blood was shed for the clove, which we think of as seasoning for pickles, the spikes in apple pie or the mask for alcoholic breath.

The discovery of America added abundantly to the jars in the apothecaries' shops—Francisco Hernández, court physician of Ferdinand II, spent seven years in Mexico and filled twenty-six volumes with drawings and observations of medicinal plants. Nicholas Monardes produced the book which became (in English edition, 1567) *Joyfull Newes out of the New Founde World.*

The additions from the Americas included *Peruvian bark* (quinine); *guaiac* (*lignum vitae,* still approved for rheumatism and for throat pastilles); ipecacuanha and the medical cure-all, *tabaco.*

The use of tobacco was popularized in Britain by Sir John Hawkins and Sir Walter Raleigh. Apart from being an indulgence, smoking was supposed to be the panacea of the North American Indian, and was regarded as especially useful as a treatment for syphilis, which was introduced into Europe about the same time. Jean Nicot, to whom we owe the word "nicotine," first saw the "miraculous herb" in Portugal, transplanted it to France and claimed that the plant was infallible. It was applied in leaf form to cancerous ulcers; used as snuff to cure headaches; as smoke to alleviate asthma; and, ritualistically, in the treatment of syphilis. This was alleged to have been the practice of the Indians of Brazil. While huge cigars were smoked over the victim as he lay on a *hammock* (which originally meant, according to some, "tobacco-bed"), tobacco leaves were applied to his sores and medicine men sucked the poison out of him.

But the apothecaries, like the pipe-indulgers, had to fight hard for the use of tobacco, against the edicts of the popes; the penalties (including nose-slitting) imposed by Moslem Sultans and Russian tsars; and James I's *Counterblaste to Tobacco.* In this he described it as "a custom loathsome to the eye, hateful to the nose, harmful to the brain, dangerous to the lungs . . . resembling the Stygian smoke in the pit that is bottomless."

3. SADDLEBAG DRUGS

The backwoods doctors, who followed the covered wagons and the iron tracks of the railroads which opened up the frontiers of America, carried their surgery and their dispensary in their saddlebags. They could ply the knife and the saw, amputate and probe. They might have ether or chloroform, if they had heard of Crawford Long, Morton or Simpson. They might use carbolic if the news of Lister and his antisepsis had reached them. But they knew little of the nature of infections or contagions because the disputations over Pasteur and Koch were far away. They relied on bleeding, cupping and leeching, and their invariable stand-bys were Dover's powder, dragon's blood, Peruvian bark, and calomel, the mercurial drug. Those were the four suits in their medical pack of cards, which they shuffled and dealt for any situation. As one doctor-on-horseback put it: He had, in his life's practice, "dispensed enough calomel to load a paddle-steamer and cupped enough blood to float it."

To quote Oliver Wendell Holmes, Sr., once again: "Will you think I am disrespectful to my profession if I ask whether, even in Massachusetts, a dose of calomel is not sometimes given by a physician on the same principle as that upon which a landlord prescribes bacon-and-eggs—because he cannot think of anything else quite so handy."

Without questioning the courage, the self-sacrifice and devotion of the pioneer doctors nor underestimating that physicians' other attribute—the giving of confidence and comfort, which is often half the battle—it is more than likely that in frontier days any medicine man or wise squaw of the Five Nations knew more medicine than the medical camp-followers of the victorious white man.

That was the great contradiction of the nineteenth century—that while the science of medicine advanced the art of medicine dragged. This was an age of great discoveries about the body and mind of man. It saw the development of organic chemistry; of physiological chemistry (biochemistry); of anesthetics; bacteriology, and with it antisepsis and asepsis; and the diagnostic identification of manifold diseases. It saw the invention of new instruments—the stethoscope, for sounding the heart and lungs;

the ophthalmoscope, for examining the eyes; the sphyg-mograph, for measuring blood pressure; the laryngoscope (invented by Garcia, a singing teacher) for studying the throat; and, at the close of the century, that great leap forward, X rays.

The nineteenth century was marked by the great advances of public health, the development of sanitation and industrial health measures and with them, what are not always fully appreciated as powerful instruments of medical discovery, vital statistics and numerical epidemiology. Great strides were made in mass medicine, if that term is taken to include the growth of the army medical services; Florence Nightingale and her nurses; the improvement of hospitals; and the courageous advance into tropical medicine. Preventive medicine, in the direct terms of vaccination, inoculation and immunology, gathered strength from the knowledge furnished by Pasteur. Protective medicine, and the science of nutrition, burgeoned at the tail end of the century. Psychology and psychiatry and the new approach to mental sickness were products of that progressive age.

Progressive? Yes, in terms of medical science, of experimental proof and precise measurements. But it was also the century of fantastic fads and professional bigotry. Phrenology, which had a basis of cerebral anatomy, became the playground of quacks and charlatans. Hydropathy, again with a rational basis, was carried to absurd lengths by the cults of Mesmerism, Temples of Health, "stroking," Odic Force, Rademacherism, Okenism (which postulated "ideally every child should be a boy") and innumerable others which exploited human credulity and valetudinarianism. Those were the days of the American Medicine Shows—of the great Phineas Barnum ("There's a sucker born every minute"); of John D. Rockefeller's father, "Doctor" William Rockefeller, who peddled patent medicines in Ohio; and the many mountebanks who ran sideshows at fairs to hawk the "elixir of life" or "snake oil" and cure-alls.

In New York alone, in 1840, over $100,000 was spent on advertising secret nostrums. And that was nothing compared with the operations of "Professor" Thomas Holloway, who used the Great Pyramid itself as a poster site for his Universal Pill and anticipated the American soft-drink companies of this century by advertising on posters and in newspapers literally from China to Peru. He died worth two million dollars and there were five other men living in London at that time who had become multimillionaires from the sale of their patent medicines— including one, a soothing syrup, which is reputed to have killed 15,000 children a year. As James Russell Lowell said: "What need of Aladdin's Lamp when we can build a palace with a patent pill?"

Just as deplorable in its way was nineteenth-century medical bigotry. If the quacks deceived the public by their irresponsibility, the qualified doctors deprived the public by their excessive "responsibility." The two were not dissociated. The doctors were so obsessed by quackery that they distrusted innovations, even when they were scientifically based. They were safe in their orthodoxy, even although their patients were not. They were as canonical in their beliefs as any clergymen and woe betide the heretic who breached the canons!

In the 1850s, Oliver Wendell Holmes (who has been so extensively invoked thus far because he was so open-minded to new truths and open-eyed to the weaknesses of his profession) fell foul of his colleagues. Or rather his colleagues fell foul of him. Holmes, with an insight which he shared with Semmelweis of Vienna, had produced, in 1843, his conclusions that childbed fever, which he called the "black-death" of mothers, was contagious. He insisted that women in childbed should not be attended by physicians who had been handling corpses, or other cases of puerperal fever, or patients with other fevers. He suggested that doctors should wash their hands in chloride of lime. This caused an uproar in a profession the respectability of which insisted that doctors should attend their cases in frock coats and cuffs. These, of course, accumulated germs, although, in fairness to the doctors, neither they nor Holmes really knew that, because Pasteur had still to come along with the evidence. Holmes was relying on observation and common sense.

Ten years later the leaders of the profession awoke to the existence of this doctrine. Hodge, professor of obstetrics at the University of Pennsylvania, begged his students to "divest their minds of the dread that they could ever carry the dreadful virus." Meigs, professor of midwifery at Jefferson Medical College, Philadelphia, scorning Holmes, said that he preferred to attribute the deaths to "accident, or providence, of which I can form no conception, rather than a contagion of which I cannot form any clear idea. ..."

Holmes replied vigorously: "There is no quarrel here between men, but there is a deadly incompatibility and exterminating warfare between doctrines. ... if I am right, let doctrines which lead to professional homicide be no longer taught from the chairs of those great institutions."

He was right and scientific proof was abundantly to confirm him and Semmelweis, who, a less resilient character than Holmes, was crushed by the antagonism of his Austrian colleagues and died in an insane asylum. But tens of thousands of mothers were yet to be sacrificed to the injured vanity of a profession.

14. ART VS. SCIENCE

Thus in the nineteenth century the science of medicine and the art of medicine were inherently in conflict. With greatly increased knowledge about the working of the human body, the practicing doctor was still using a trained intuition and an age-old inheritance of drugs; treating symptoms and rarely causes of disease. But, at least, he regarded his patient as a familiar and not just as "a case," impersonalized by the findings of the pathological laboratory or the shadowgraph.

Not until the middle 1930s was the doctor to have the ammunition with which to snipe at a particular germ or strain of germs. Today, with the sulfa drugs, the antibiotics and their permutations and combinations, he has a whole arsenal. Although the *materia medica* of the traditional pharmacist still remains, over 80 per cent of prescriptions now written by doctors are for drugs which did not exist twenty years ago.

There are those who would say that perhaps medicine has become too much of a science and has diminished as an essential art; that there is too much specialization and too little comprehending of the whole man, and that Lord Horder was right in preferring to see the captain, rather than the radio operator, on the bridge.

Part Two

DEMONS, DEMIGODS, AND DOCTORS

> Then the medicine-men, the Medas,
> The magicians, the Wabenos,
> And the Jossakeeds, the prophets,
> Came to visit Hiawatha;
> Built a Sacred Lodge beside him,
> To appease him, to console him,
> Walked in silent, grave procession,
> Bearing each a pouch of healing,
> Skin of beaver, lynx, or otter,
> Filled with magic roots and simples,
> Filled with very potent medicines,
>   When he heard their steps approach-
>   ing,
> Hiawatha ceased lamenting,
> Called no more on Chibiabos . . .
>
> —HENRY WADSWORTH LONGFELLOW
> *Hiawatha*

1. THE HEALING INSTINCT

The instinct to heal and to cure exists even in the lower animals. The owl rids herself of feather lice by taking dust baths. A wounded animal will lick its wounds, using the germ-killing qualities of its spittle. A creature suffering from a deficiency disease will trek great distances to find a salt lake or vegetation containing the trace elements it lacks. Medicinal spas, for human purposes, have been found because they were the instinctive haunts of animals seeking curative baths or purgative waters.

Such instincts are deep and sometimes shrewder than the medical textbooks. Sheep with a diet deficient in lime have been known to eat, with geometrical exactitude, the grass of a squared plot which had been limed, before turning to other pastures which would satisfy their hunger but lacked the subtler medical requirements. On the South African veldt, cattle were dying of a mysterious epidemic. One group survived and it was found that they were eating the bark and herbage of a tree in the trunk of which there was a single copper nail. The rest of the cattle were sick from a deficiency of minute traces of copper.

Such instincts to find healing sources are just as real as those which tell a creature, animal, bird or insect how to find, or differentiate, its food—distinguishing what is nutritive from what is poisonous. And such uncomplicated and intuitive healing is part of man's heritage from his animal ancestry.

2. SCALPEL-MAKING ANIMAL

The simplest definition of man was that given by Benjamin Franklin—a "toolmaking animal." This may not seem particularly flattering to the intellect which can release energy from the atom. But if one analyzes Franklin's description, its essential truth is obvious. Our kinsfolk, the apes, and the tea-party chimpanzees, have obviously a degree of intelligence, but they do not make tools. To make them needs imagination and to apply them needs not only finger skills but intellectual capacity—the power to reason as well as to react or to imitate.

If we are, then, to determine when man first took an active, as distinct from an intuitive, interest in medicine, we have to think of him first as a tool-using surgeon. As earliest man did not have the foresight to provide his posterity with copies of his clinical prescriptions, we can deduce his knowledge only from his tools—from the "celts" or sharp flints he left, and from the uses to which he put them. It would be sheer guesswork to assume that he anticipated later doctors, or "leeches," by opening veins and practicing bloodletting. Since flesh and organs do not survive in prehistoric remains, there is no evidence. What have remained are skeletons and these provide significant information.

The Ape Man, the Near Man, or the Dawn Man, may all have had some medical or surgical practices, but there is little or no trace of them. We can, with more confidence, go back 30,000 years to the types who were recognizably man in physiognomy and posture. In the prehistoric skulls which have been collected in all parts of the world

—including Peru—are to be found the holes made by the trephiners. These are holes cut out of the bone with flint instruments to obtain access to the brain. That the actual operation was carried out on living "patients" and that they survived is evident from the rounded edges showing that the bone had grown again after the operation. This operation still persists in modern surgery and among primitive people throughout the world today. It has been practiced throughout the ages. The interesting question is how prehistoric man came to perform it and for what purposes. Since the only "case books" are the skulls themselves we can merely speculate.

How they arrived at trephining at all can be reasonably assumed. The one thing which prehistoric man would know about himself would be the nature of his skeleton. That would remain as the proof of his kind when the flesh had vanished and would be recognizably different from the bone remains of other animals. He would recognize his own chassis. Of that framework only one part would be apparent as a container—the casket of the brain box, or skull. If in the living being that casket could be opened "something" could be released. What was that "something"? Was it a demon who afflicted the victims? Or was there a surgical motive to release an identified pain? We know from contemporary primitives that it could have been both or either. And it would appear from the evidence of the Stone Age skulls of thousands of years ago that it could have been treatment for a localized condition—migraine, epilepsy or even brain tumors. The positioning of some holes would indicate that.

Indeed it is profitless diversion to try to distinguish between ritualistic and therapeutic trephining, since in any primitive society, contemporary or prehistoric, the roles of the priest and the medicine man were inseparable. In the cave of the Trois Frères in France there is the famous wall drawing, reputedly 16,000 years old, which shows the medicine man with a "stag mask" and in the caves of Altamira in Spain, probably 20,000 years old, are found the wonderful cave pictures of bison and other animals uncannily exact in anatomical detail. Occasionally one finds, in wall paintings made by prehistoric man, the spears or arrows plunged exactly into the vital organs of the animals, showing that in terms of their animal victims, if not of themselves, prehistoric hunters had a pre-

cise knowledge of anatomy. Neither the Stag Man nor the
bison is likely to have been drawn merely as a form of
artistic expression. For one thing the cave pictures were
drawn in awkward places and by the light of stone lamps,
with animal fats as fuel. They were probably themselves
ritualistic. The arrow in the heart was not just a textbook
illustration to instruct hunters but a piece of artistic sorcery to ensure good hunting.

The Stag Man of Trois Frères, the earliest doctor we can
find, is the prototype of the bilbo, witch doctor, medicine
man or shaman of every primitive society from neolithic
times to the present day and, in geographic range, from
the North American Indians to the Polynesians. This extraordinary consistency in magic and folklore throughout
the ages and throughout the world, diversified by time and
remote in distance, shows that the essential traits of folk
medicine and ancient medicine have been alike in tendency and have differed only in unimportant details. This
is understandable because people struggling with pain and
affliction would everywhere arrive at similar supernatural conclusions.

When man developed imagination, he became aware
of the intangible forces which beset him—the loud-voiced
thunder, the terrifying lightning (from which, setting fire
to a forest, man probably first captured fire), earthquakes,
volcanic eruptions, eclipses, the auroras, the moving shad-
ows cast by the sun or his reflection in water. To these
natural phenomena his imagination gave supernatural
meanings. He identified them with gods, or demons or
spirits. He came to worship the sun, the moon, the stars,
trees, rivers, springs, fire, winds and the animals which he
feared. His religion was animistic—believing that his
world swarmed with invisible spirits which brought, among
other things, disaster, disease and death.

As he advanced, he grasped the intangibles, in the
sense that he represented them as carvings, symbols with
which he could cope more easily than with the invisible
forces which they represented. So he moved from nature
worship to fetish worship. A disease was (and is) regarded by primitive peoples as the work of demons who
had to be placated by sacrifices or cajoled by offerings.
A further stage was an association of ideas which led him
to attribute his afflictions to a human enemy working by
spells and sorcery (as in African ju-ju), to be combated

by similar witchcraft. Yet a further development was a belief in a hereafter populated by spirits of the dead, among whom were offended ghosts who would take revenge on the living in the form of disease.

3. PAGAN PSYCHIATRY

Everywhere, no matter how far separated by time or distance, the common feature of the witch doctor is his practice of assuming a terrifying aspect, covering himself with skins of animals so as to resemble an enormous beast walking on its hind legs, shouting, raving, going into trances, or making magical movements or signs. Such practices may seem grotesque, but they are not as absurd as they appear.

Take it purely ritualistically: If you regard the enemy (the demon causing disease) as something grotesque and ugly, you confront it with something equally so. The garb provides the confidence of the pretense. Moreover, where animals become vested with the supernatural, their skins are the "external soul" and always, everywhere, men have "protected" themselves magically by wearing skins. Hercules practiced preventive medicine when he wore the skin of a lion, the totem of his tribe, the Heraclidae. The priests of Babylon conducted rituals in fishskins.

Another object of "dressing-up" and of the ostentatious magic of the witch doctor is to impress the patient, and to give any practical treatment an awesome authority. All the abracadabra and conjuring is not only to impress the gods but also to induce the right frame of mind in the patient.

Moreover a great deal of useful medical treatment goes into witch-doctoring. It is too easy to dismiss the herbals, the concoctions, the poultices, and the "physical therapy" as the tricks of primitive mountebanks. That is something which modern medical science has to remember when, with its arrogant confidence in its new drugs and methods, it seeks to sweep away age-old practices. Much of it may be discarded as worthless but, as I have argued with Western-trained doctors in the East, to discard all of it may sometimes be a case of "throwing out the baby with the bath water"—losing medical virtues of permanent value.

One common practice of medicine men is to try to extract the active cause of a disease by sucking it through a hollow tube, sometimes symbolically and sometimes actually, and spitting out the poison. The identification with animals has also a deeper medical-biological significance: The totem, the identification of people with an animal symbol, is universal—it exists in the coats-of-arms of noble families—and in its origin is eugenic. People of the same totem cannot marry—a simple taboo on incest and inbreeding. In some cases eating the totem animal is part of a healing rite. Certain organs of certain animals are regarded as the seats of the spirits—the heart, the liver, and the brain. If eaten raw they are supposed to be powerful therapeutics. On the other hand, the eating of certain organs, e.g., polar bear liver in the case of the Eskimo, may be ritually forbidden for excellent medical reasons. This eating of organs to treat similar organs in the patient—isotherapy (like-curing-like)—persisted in the sacrificial rituals of the Romans and the Greeks and was still extant in the pharmacopoeias of Western Europe as late as the eighteenth century. In religious rituals they have become the sacrificial cakes and sacramental wine (body and blood).

The cult and the art of the witch doctor and the medicine man have never been entirely limited to the supernatural. These men acquired a primitive science, learning from experience and accumulated tradition certain reliable practices. They advanced herb-doctoring, bonesetting, surgery and midwifery in difficult confinements.

Just as food husbandry grew from the observation that certain plants and grains were good to eat and could be deliberately cultivated, so the medicine man and wise woman observed the nature of illnesses and herbals and other treatments which were food for them and passed on their confirmed experience to other generations. The hieratic writings of the Egyptian papyri reveal an extensive *materia medica*. Homeric poems are a medical source book. The Ancient Egyptians, Chinese and Aztecs had botanic gardens. The virtues as well as the lethal qualities of poisons were early discovered. Ipecacuanha, the Amazonian poison which is also an emetic, has already been mentioned. *Curare* was another arrow poison, which killed by paralyzing the muscles and which, in our generation, has, in discreet doses, become a valuable help to the surgeon in his operation techniques.

Mandrake root is another example of a plant the qualities of which have been known to—and variously interpreted by—many widely separated peoples. The *Mandragora* has large, bifurcated taproots which are supposed to resemble human legs and to give the plant the appearance of a manikin. Folklore has attributed to it animal properties: it was supposed to scream when uprooted, and anyone who heard it scream would go mad. Magical virtues were attributed to it. It was believed to be an aphrodisiac and to cure barrenness. When Rachel asked her sister Leah for mandrakes (Genesis xxx:14) it was to enable her to bear children. She would have been wise also to use them in giving birth to those children, because mandrake has genuine narcotic values. The Egyptians regarded it as the special gift of Ra, the sun-god. Dioscorides used it as an anesthetic for surgical operations in the ninth century. Its narcotic effects were hymned by Shakespeare in *Antony and Cleopatra:*

> Give me to drink mandragora. . . .
> That I might sleep out this great gap of time
> My Antony is away.

Practically all peoples everywhere have had their narcotics—opium, hashish, hemp, coca, and many more. And there is a universality in the use of indigenous herbals to serve as abortifacients to limit families.

When, in the story of the Nativity, we recall the Three Wise Men who brought to the stable the gifts of gold, frankincense and myrrh, we are reminded of the spices which came out of the East. But this was not only ritual incense. Frankincense is *olibanum*, a gum resin which is still prescribed for women's complaints and for chest and throat affections. Myrrh provides a stimulant and an astringent. It is used in chronic bronchitis and, again, in women's complaints. *Tincture of myrrh* is applied for toothache and gumboils.

At the Crucifixion (Mark xv:23) it is written: "And they gave him to drink wine, mingled with myrrh: but he received it not." For the preparation and preservation of the body of Jesus (John xix:39) Nicodemus brought myrrh and aloes about an hundred pounds.

4. SUMERIAN MEDICINE

In the beginnings of medicine, diseases were visitations —the whims or revenge of affronted gods or spirits, as unpredictable as the elements. The priest and the physician were one and the same. What man might damage, men might try to repair—stanch the wound, rough-set a broken limb, or manipulate a dislocated joint—but, in early and right up to recent times, the surgeon was just the rude mechanic in the caste system of medicine.

In that graveyard of lost civilizations, in the region which is now called Mesopotamia or, on the map, Iraq, city cultures existed 5000 years ago. While the predynastic Egyptians were still working with flints, the Sumerians had already advanced to fine metals and delicate craftsmanship and to a prosperity which came from trade and a long-established craft tradition.

Before the Flood, and long before Abraham left Ur to become the Biblical Patriarch, there existed at Ur a culture with delicate painted pottery which preceded even the Sumerians. It had settled and grown on the rich alluvial silt brought down by the Euphrates. It has long been agreed that the story of the Flood as told in Genesis is based on the Sumerian legend of which the oldest written versions date from at least 2000 B.C. But in 1929 Sir Leonard Woolley found proofs of the Flood. He had been excavating the graves of the kings and had been convinced that the advanced civilization which they represented must have had a long past behind it. So he sank his shafts deeper through buried rubbish until he reached clean clay, uniform throughout and of a texture which showed that it had been laid there by water. The Arab workmen insisted that this was the bottom of everything —the river silt on which the original settlement had been built, but Woolley did not believe it. The stratum was too high above what had been the original marsh. So he set them digging again and they cut through eight feet of clay and found themselves in an even older culture. This was the Ur which had been drowned by the Flood, overwhelmed by the waters as Herculaneum was engulfed by lava. A flood capable of depositing eight feet of clay must have been a mighty one—enough to convince those who survived that the whole world had been engulfed. The date must have been not later than 2700 B.C.

The Chaldeans of Ur were a remarkable people, the founders of astronomy as an exact science. A thousand years before Christ, Chaldean astronomers calculated the length of the year as 365 days, 6 hours, 15 minutes and 41 seconds—a measurement which our modern precision instruments have corrected by only 26 minutes 26 seconds. The measurements of the diameter of the moon were more accurate than those of Copernicus, whom we accept as the founder of modern astronomy.

In the Royal Tombs of Ur, excavated by Woolley, apart from the wealth buried there, was found evidence of living sacrifice. When the royal personage died, his, or her, retinue followed to the Hereafter. They marched down a sloping ramp into the death pits and were buried alive.

In a pit 37 feet by 24 feet were found the bodies of six men servants and sixty-eight women. The bodies were disposed in rows across the floor and there was evidence in the neat arrangement of the skeletons that there had been no violence and no terror. Many of the women wore headdresses which were found in good order and undisturbed except by the pressure of the earth. That could not have been so if they had been knocked on the head or stabbed or had suffered the agonies of suffocation. The evidence is all against their having been killed outside the pits and in favor of voluntary sacrifice.

If, therefore, a coroner's inquest were carried out on those eloquent bones of 4500 years ago, the verdict would be that the courtiers chose to die with their king and queen and that they drank some powerful sleeping draught and composed themselves to sleep. Some attendant descended into the pit and with gentle care arranged harps on the breast and the gold leaves of the headgear before the pit was filled in with earth.

If we accept the evidence of the soporifics and of the cosmetics in the queen's death chamber at Ur, we can assume also that the Sumerians of Erech, Ur, Kish and Lagash had a system of healing drugs as well. Many small copper knives have been dug up which would suggest that they were used by surgeons as scalpels. From Kish came a pictographic script of about 4200 B.C., and from the same site came tablets bearing on medicine. From

Lagash came a physician's seal of about 3000 B.C. Such seals were engraved on cylinders which were rolled in the wet clay and used as signatures for the tiles which were the records of the times. This one showed Iru, a god regarded as a form, or incarnation, of Nergal, the god of pestilence and disease. These records also show that drains existed at Kish as early as 3000 B.C.

5. ASSYRO-BABYLONIAN MEDICINE

The Sumerian civilization came to an end about 2000 B.C. and was replaced by the Assyro-Babylonian. As in all early civilizations, the roles of the priest and physician were inseparable. This had to be so because the priesthood was the continuity, and repository, of accumulated and associated ideas and knowledge. Facts were observed, even if they were imperfectly understood, and the medicinal effects of, for example, desert herbs, or of resins exuded by shrubs during the summer heat, would be noted and passed on as priestly lore. Just as astronomy, as an exact and rational science, became the magic of astrology, so factual observations of conditions and treatments became the stage props of priestly ritual. The two —astrology and medicine—were intermingled.

King Ashurbanipal of Assyria (669-626 B.C.) collected in the great library of Nineveh over 30,000 clay tablets, of which 800 were medical. From these it is apparent that demons were held to be the cause of disease. Diagnosis was based on simple inspection of the patient. His or her prospects were decided by divination and augury by examination of the liver of a sheep into the nostrils of which the patient had breathed and so transferred his symptoms. Or the priests read meanings into blood drawn from the patient, or specimens of his urine or saliva. From this ritualism much substantial knowledge must have been gained. The Babylonians had a knowledge of the structure of the liver which was preserved in exact clay models —far better specimens of anatomical illustration than the imperfect and misleading conceptions of the liver that persisted through the Middle Ages.

The lists of medicaments and the prescriptions and treatments used by the priest-doctors of Babylonia are extensive. They are mixed up with incantations and charms, and what would be a genuine remedy even today was compounded with some revolting ingredient, intended to disgust the demon. For example, sore eyes were, and are still, common in the lands of the khamsin, the hot dry wind which blows out of the Arabian desert. The eye trouble was ascribed to the Demon of the Southwest wind, the image for which was a dog-headed eagle with lion's claws. The wind was supposed to be frightened by the ugliness of his own image, which, accordingly, was set up outside the houses to keep him and his afflictions away. To treat sore eyes, the priest-doctor would prescribe cutting up an onion and mixing it and drinking it with beer. This was obviously to encourage tears, with (as we now know) their germicidal properties. Then the eyes were to be assuaged with oil. So far this is commendable treatment but, by priestly reckoning, not drastic enough against such a nasty demon. So to the straightforward prescription was added the ritualistic one: "Thou shalt disembowel a yellow frog, mix its gall in curd and apply to the eye."

Nergal, the Babylonian god of disease who was adopted by the Assyro-Phoenicians as Beelzebub, their chief god, had as his symbol the fly. The implication is obvious—those ancients recognized that insects were carriers of disease. The outstanding achievement of the Assyro-Babylonians in public hygiene was their recognition of the transmission of leprosy. Fearing the contagion, they expelled the leper from the community: "Nevermore shall he know the ways of his abiding place," says an inscription over 3500 years old.

It would appear that while the priestly class, the *ashipu,* were concerned with inner medicine, there were also surgeons (strange how this discrimination between physician and surgeon repeats itself all through history). These were the practical doctors, the *asu,* who dealt with wounds, visible sores, fractures and snakebites. They were also skilled in herbal and mineral cures.

By the time of Hammurabi, the great king, (1948-1905 B.C.) they were recognized and esteemed as a non-priestly medical profession. While the priests were answerable to the gods, the *asu* were answerable to the state. Their practices were controlled by governmental regulation.

Among the regulations laid down by the Code of Hammurabi were those governing fees (and penalties) for the non-priestly doctor.

"If the doctor shall treat a gentleman and shall open an abscess with a bronze knife or shall preserve the eye of the patient, he shall receive ten shekels of silver. If the patient be a freeman he shall pay five shekels. If the patient be a slave, the owner shall pay two shekels."

But woe betide the *asu* who failed! If in opening the abscess he killed the patient, or if he destroyed the sight of the eye, his hands were cut off. That did not apply in the case of a slave. If he killed or damaged the eyesight of a slave, he had to give the master a new slave, or, in the case of one eye, pay half the cost of a new slave. There was no margin for error.

There was a stage of development of Babylonian medicine which has been described by Herodotus and might be called "shared diagnosis." According to Herodotus: "They bring their sick into the market place. Then those who pass by the sick person confer with him about the disease to discover whether they have ever been afflicted with the same disease and advise him to have recourse to the same treatment as that by which they themselves, or others they have known, have been cured. And they are not allowed to pass by a sick person in silence, without inquiring the nature of his distemper."

If we think of this as primitive, let us remember that customs die hard! Think of our friends who inflict their symptoms on us and all the conflicting advice we offer in return. For "Babylonian market place" read "sewing bee" or "country club."

6. VEDANTIC MEDICINE

Evidence suggests that, after the Flood, which swamped Ur, the later Sumerians came from the East: "And it came to pass that as they journeyed from the east, they came upon a plain in the land of Shinar" (which is Babylon) "and they dwelt there" (Gen. xi:2). Another Sumerian legend implies that the "replacements" came by sea, from the south. Either would be consistent with the Aryan-Dravidian movement from India, bringing with them a knowledge of agriculture, metalworking, the potter's wheel, and writing.

This is not the occasion to argue where city cultures

riginated but to realize that thousands of years ago peoples in many parts of the world were struggling towards a practice which we call medicine.

The Vedantic or Vedic medicine of India goes back, in written form, to the *Rig Veda* of 1500 B.C. and the *Atharva Veda*. They reveal a medicine entirely god-ridden, with incantations and spells to appease the demons of disease or the human ill-wishers who conspired black magic. It was witchcraft and wizardry.

In the Brahminical period (800 B.C. to 1000 A.D.) medicine was entirely in the hands of priests and scholars, with a medical school at Benares. In 300 B.C. hospitals were in existence and surgery, in which the ancient Hindus excelled, was flowering. Yet, with the sort of confusion we will find again in the Middle Ages, the priestly domination confused the knowledge of the human body and the concepts of anatomy were weird and wonderful.

Yet there was an insight among the practitioners which anticipated discoveries medical science is only now making. In the *Susruta* (fifth century A.D.) we find the basis of modern plastic surgery. This, among the ancient Hindus, was used as "rhinoplasty," which means turning down a flap of the skin of the forehead to repair unsightly nose defects. This was rather more than the cosmetic improvement of the tip-tilt of a film actress, because, in those days, infidelity in a wife was punished by cutting off her nose, and the surgeons devised this operation to repair the mutilation. What is interesting is this early recognition of modern immunology (which means a great deal more, nowadays, than vaccination or inoculation). With our present-day knowledge of genetics, we know that the body-system rejects alien cells. So, if an attempt is made to graft a piece of skin or flesh from someone else, the body will discard the patch. Only like will repair like—a graft must come from the person of the patient (although a graft from an identical twin will "take"). The ancients knew this and used the flap method—a patch from the person, nourished by the person's own blood supply.

The *Susruta* described 121 surgical instruments—scalpels, lancets, saws, scissors, needles, hooks, probes, detectors, forceps, catheters, syringes, bougies, and so forth. The one operative process which the Hindus did not know was ligaturing—the method of tying the end of a blood vessel. When they skillfully amputated limbs, they checked the blood by cautery or boiling oil or pressure. They "cut for stone" more than a thousand years before Oliver Wendell Holmes's "wandering friar." They delivered babies by Caesarean section. They used drugs, like belladonna and Indian hemp, as operational anesthetics. They developed bamboo splints and efficiently set fractures.

They were highly advanced in diagnostic methods. The *Susruta* divides 1120 diseases into "natural" and "supernatural," and teaches palpation (feeling with the hand and fingers for anything abnormal) and auscultation (listening for sounds within the body) of the heart, lungs and womb. It gives a recognizable description of malarial fever and attributes it to the mosquitoes, while other Sanskrit literature of ancient origin recognizes rats as the carriers of plague, describes diabetes, and recommends inoculation against smallpox.

Indian medicaments were, in those remote times, remarkable for their range and value. The *Susruta* lists 760 medicinal plants, many of which came into the pharmacopeia of the West and are still there. Emphasis was laid on aphrodisiacs and the recognition of poisons, with antidotes for snake bite and other poisonous bites. There is a regular hymn of praise for garlic, which we have tended to regard as the appetizer of the Latin races but are now discovering to have special virtues in the discouragement of gastric ulcers.

Even more significant today is the Hindu drug *rauwolfia*, from the leaves of a plant of the Himalayan foothills. Age-old in its use, it was a "tranquilizer"; it quietened what we would call "nerves." Whenever Mahatma Gandhi was under the stress of the modern world, rauwolfia would restore his philosophic detachment. Modern medical science, having extracted the active principle, now applies it in hypertension, high blood pressure, and as a treatment for mental cases. Thus the Old World—"old" both in time and distance—is redressing the stresses of our New World, of modern tensions.

7. PERSIAN MEDICINE

Persian medicine has an Aryan tradition common with that of India. The main influence it exercised on medical history was through the cult of Zoroaster (1000 B.C.) and y giving us the word "drug" itself. "Drug" did not mean medicament but a demon. Its inversion to our sense of he term is rather like the Babylonians' use of images of he evil gods to frighten away the gods themselves. Or like he "sympathetic medicine" of the Middle Ages (and even ater), which treated the spear which caused the wound ather than the wound itself. So, in practice, a "drug" vas the incantation and the medicament against the)rug, or demon.

The important principle of Zoroaster was that the elements—air, fire, water and earth—were pure and must ot be defiled, and so this religion brought to medicine he cult of cleanliness and ritual directions against uncleanliness, which had striking similarities to the Hebrew ode of Leviticus.

Ahru-Mazda, the All-knowing One, the good god, had, s his sixteenth name, "The Healing One," and his inunctions were: *"One may heal with holiness; one may eal with the law; one may heal with the knife; one may eal with herbs; one may heal with Thy Holy Word, which ; the best-healing of all remedies."*

The priests were the *Magi* (hence "magic") and they vere those who conjured out the evil demons. But there vere also practitioners of the medical and surgical skills njoined by Ahru-Mazda. The competence of the candidate was tested by letting him practice on heretics. If hree died in succession, he was regarded as unfit and was isqualified by the risk—which no one was likely to take —that the loss of any further patient would be treated as remeditated murder. (This rule was tough not only on he heretics but on any aspiring medico, because religion barred him from any experimental training in anatomy. A corpse was unclean and therefore the faithful could not andle it.) But if all three heretics recovered, he had qualfied and subsequent deaths of patients were merely proessional mishaps and not capital offenses.

Apart from hygiene, derived from cult-cleanliness, the ncient Persians added considerably to the knowledge of rugs and plants. And, being at the watershed of East nd West, they influenced not only later developments hroughout the Middle East but Chinese medicine as well.

8. CHINESE MEDICINE

Before turning back to the Middle East, it would be profitable to look at the medicine of China, because, as we shall see, the development of medical knowledge was a sort of lend-lease—a giving and a taking—between many cultures.

The Emperor Shen Nung (2737 B.C.) is regarded as the founder of Chinese medicine. To him is attributed *Pentsao* (The Great Herbal) and to the Emperor Huang-ti (2697 B.C.) is credited *Neiching* (The Canon of Medicine). Those books were written in lacquer on strips of bamboo. The ideogram for "physician" was, like the Egyptian hieroglyph, a lancet in the upper half and a bleeding-glass in the lower.

In the *Neiching* it is written: "All the blood of the body is under the control of the heart and flows in a continuous circle and never stops." That was 4300 years before William Harvey's discovery of the circulation of the blood In *Neiching,* the physiology is picturesque: The heart is the king; the lungs are his executives; the liver, his general; the gall-bladder his attorney general, and the spleen his steward, who supervises the five tastes, and the "three burning spaces"—the thorax, the abdomen and the pelvis —and is responsible for the sewage system of the body.

From the Chow Dynasty (1123-256 B.C.) onwards the literature includes works on the blood system and the intestines, with reliable studies of the physical nature of the organs. And it was in this period that the tradition of Chinese fee-paying by results was established.

In *The Golden Mirrors of Medicine,* an encyclopedia produced in forty volumes under the instructions of the Emperor Kien Lung (1644 A.D.) the centuries of medical knowledge were marshaled and accounts given of a great many methods of treatment, including massage, manipulative surgery and acupuncture. Acupuncture, since it involved sticking needles into 365 specified points in the body, gave ancient Chinese medicine its exceptional knowledge of anatomy and anthropometric measurements the accuracy of which cannot be improved upon today The Chinese also introduced fingerprinting, knew about preventive inoculation for smallpox, and had a system of vital statistics, introduced in 1105 B.C.

The range of drugs and herbals was immense. They probably anticipated Paracelsus by centuries in the use of mercury in the treatment of venereal disease, of which gonorrhea was identified in 2500 B.C. and syphilis was noted in the Ming Dynasty in the fourteenth century A.D. Many of the medicines seem weird, fanciful or revolting to Western (modern) minds. But we are barely a century removed from similar "abominations" here, and it is always necessary to repeat that medical science cannot afford to be supercilious and should not discard age-old practices until they have been scientifically examined.

To the instance of the Indian *rauwolfia,* already mentioned, might be added the "witchcraft" of the Chinese in preparing concoctions of toadskins, as a treatment for dropsy. We now know why. The virtue of toadskin lies in its richness in *bufagin,* which produces a free flow of urine, so helping to drain the tissues, and in *adrenalin,* which slows down the heart rate, increases the blood pressure, and speeds the excretion of sugar.

The Chinese have another claim to distinction—that of being the advance guard of forensic medicine. About 1241 A.D., during the Sung Dynasty, there was produced the *Hsi Yuan Lu,* being instructions to coroners, giving minute directions for the examination of a corpse, on death or after exhumation. Apart from the details of how to produce evidence of blows, stabbings, stranglings and poisons, and distinguishing between murders and suicides, it also gives instructions for artificial respiration and antidotes for poisons.

2. *EGYPTIAN MEDICINE*

When the new-fledged doctor, fresh from his course in twentieth-century medical science, examines his first patient and writes his first prescription, he avows himself a neophyte of a pagan, magical cult. He may not know it as he scribbles his instructions to dispense the latest antibiotic or the newest sulfa drug. But, at the top of his prescription, he writes ℞ —just a Roman "R" with a stroke through the foot—and in this act he invokes Horus, the bird-headed god of the Egyptians. It is modern science reinsuring itself!

Of course, as a rational being, he will probably deny it. He will say that it is no more than the dog-latin of the medico—"R" for *Recipe*, meaning "Take," just like the cook's "recipe": "Take four eggs. . . ." No, sir! As Sir William Osler pointed out, it is the "Eye of Horus," the Egyptian amulet dating back 5000 years.

Horus was the son of Isis and Osiris, who avenged the murder of Osiris by Seth. In the course of the struggle Seth plucked out the eye of Horus, before he was mastered by him. Isis called in Thoth, the god of wisdom, who restored the missing eye. By virtue of his suffering, in filial devotion, Horus became the god of healing and his eye the protecting device.

In origin the amulet was like this:

During Roman times, Galen (130-200 A.D.) advised his fellow physicians to sprinkle their writings with Egyptian symbols to impress their patients, and one of those symbols was the Eye of Horus. At first it depicted two eyes, which became corrupted into two Roman "Rs," back to back, like this ℟℞ and later one ℞ sufficed. This was modified during the Middle Ages into a kind of "Z," like this ⃗, which was the sign of Zeus, or Jupiter, and this, in turn, was rationalized back to ℞ and *Recipe*.

Like the sacred snake of Aesculapius, the crest of the physician, this is a reminder that modern medicine is the heir to a long tradition of myth and magic. And the influence of Ancient Egypt was immense.

In the IIIrd Dynasty, about 3000 B.C., the first pyramid was built. The Step Pyramid, at Memphis, a massive structure, rising in six unequal stages to the height of 204 feet, was built for King Zoser, by his architect, Imhotep.

But, through the centuries, the Egyptians esteemed Imhotep, not as the pyramid builder, but as a doctor. His name signified "He who cometh in peace." He was deified as the god of healing and was later identified by the Greeks with their own god of healing, Aesculapius.

As elsewhere in early times, the Egyptian priest and the physician were one and the same. Disease was a hostile orce which belonged to the invisible world. It was a malignant god or spirit, or the soul of a dead man seeking revenge on the living. When it entered into the living body, it began to break the bones, suck the marrow, drink the blood, gnaw the intestines and the heart, and devour the flesh. The duty of the priest-physician was to drive out the demon or destroy it within. To do this, he must first discover the nature of the spirit in possession and its name, and then devise the powerful magic in the form of incantations and amulets which would overcome it. Only then did he use medicine to repair the damage and restore the body.

All true medical knowledge was revealed by the gods and had been sealed by Thoth, the healer of Horus, in secret books to which only the priests could have access. Thus all medical training was concentrated in the temples. In the later dynasties, however, specialization was developed to an exceptional degree. The pharaohs surrounded themselves with physicians, each dedicated to a special organ or function. Sometimes there would be a "Guardian of the Right Eye" as well as a "Guardian of the Left Eye." The physician Irj (2500 B.C.) is described in his tomb as "The Shepherd of the Royal Anus." One of the important posts was "Skull-opener to the Pharaoh." This was the trephiner, who, when all else had failed, would open the cranium to release the demon, or, more often, the spirit of the king himself.

Women were admitted as doctors in Egypt. In the Vth Dynasty, about 2730 B.C., a tablet describes a woman as "Chief Physician," and in the later Middle Kingdom women took prominent places in the profession.

A succession of medical papyri, with hieratic texts has been found. ("Hieratic" was a sort of priestly shorthand form of the more elaborate hieroglyphic script.) The Edwin Smith Papyrus, discovered at Thebes in 1862 and presented to the New York Historical Society, relates to the period of 1600 B.C. This was a roll fifteen feet long and written on both sides. Amongst a lot of hocus-pocus, such as incantations against pestilential winds (climatic, not flatulent) and for the rejuvenation of old men, there are case histories, giving a provisional diagnosis, details of examination, prognosis (what the chances were) and treatment.

The Ebers Papyrus (about 1500 B.C.) consists of a

comprehensive collection of prescriptions for a large num
ber of ailments, and shows that while charms and ritual
still persisted there was much such medical examination
going on. The list of drugs was long and included many
which are still valued in medical practice. But the ad
vance of clinical medicine was restricted throughout th
centuries because the Book of Thoth was the orthodox
which had to be observed and physicians risked grav
penalties if they departed from it. Surgery was very primi
tive but the public health measures were often of a high
order. With our sense of hygiene (and smell) we woul
certainly have been less affronted by the conditions in an
cient Egypt than we would have been by the royal palace
of medieval Europe.

What makes Ancient Egypt especially significant t
medical study nowadays is the pictograms and bas-relief
which enable us to recognize familiar complaints (e.g.
poliomyelitis in the XVIIIth Dynasty, 1580 B.C.). And
of course, the mummies which have preserved identifi
able diseases—loin abscesses, thickening of the arteries
dental caries, gallstones and even skin eruptions.

Mummifying was not the work of the priest-doctors
who belonged to the House of Life. The House of Death
was another realm, but embalming did in fact teach much
about the organs of the body.

Let Herodotus tell the story of embalming:

"There are a set of men in Egypt who practice the ar
of embalming and make it their proper business. These
persons, when a body is brought to them, show the mourn
ers various models of corpses made in wood and painted
so as to resemble nature. The most perfect is said to b
after the manner of him, whom I do not think it is religiou
to name. The second sort is inferior to the first and les
costly and the third is cheapest of all. The bearers tel
them which model they want and conclude the bargain.

"The mode of embalming, according to the most per
fect process, is as follows: They first take a crooked piec
of iron and with it draw out the brain through the nostril
and clear the rest of the skull with drugs. Next the
make a cut along the flank with a sharp Ethiopian ston
and take out the contents of the abdomen, which the
wash thoroughly with palm wine and with repeated in
fusions of pounded aromatics. After this they fill the cav
ty with the purest bruised myrrh, with cassia and ever

kind of spices except frankincense and sew up the opening. Then the body is placed in carbonate of soda for seventy days. At the end of that time, which must not be exceeded, the body is washed and wrapped around from head to foot with bandages of fine linen cloth, smeared with gum and given back to the relatives to be encased. Such is the most costly way of embalming the dead."

Sometimes the strips of linen were 1000 yards long, and comparable with modern gauzes. There is not a single method of bandaging employed today that is not represented in the techniques of swathing the mummies.

The other methods were more cheap-jack and did no more than preserve the skin and bones.

10. MOSAIC MEDICINE

Moses, as the adopted son of Pharaoh's daughter, was in all probability trained for the priesthood, and so acquired a knowledge of hygiene and medicine. His religion —the monotheism of the Jews—did not accept the gods of disease and healing, nor the exorcism, nor the astrology, nor the incantations. God was the supreme healer as well as the source of afflictions. The Hebrew priests and prophets might heal according to the powers that God gave them.

That is why ancient Jewish medicine was mainly significant for the Mosaic Law. The priests were not physicians but medical officers of health. They were remarkably aware of communicable disease. The Book of Leviticus is an excellent sanitary code, giving instruction on proper and improper food; clean and unclean objects; the hygiene of childbirth and menstruation; and the prevention of contagion. The transmission of leprosy was recognized and directions were given for the isolation of people with infections and for the disinfection of their property. What may now be regarded as ritualistic, like the banning of pig meat, certainly had sound medical origins; pigs can cause trichinosis by passing on, in pork, threadlike worms which proliferate with serious consequences in humans. There were no doubt just as valid contemporary reasons for the banning of other creatures as food.

The nature of contagion was recognized and in Jewish cities the *shofar,* the ram's horn, was blown as a curfew warning that infection was around.

In the secular sense, therefore, the great contribution of the Jews to medicine, through the Bible and the Talmud, was in hygiene and public health measures. There was, however, another contribution which did not become apparent until later when, in the stream of Arab medicine, the Jews came to play their part as physicians and surgeons in the Middle Ages. With the ban of the Church (as we shall see) on the proper study of anatomy, the wandering Jew, having picked up Greek Hippocratic medicine as well as Arab medical learning, had the information deriving from *kosher* and *terephah*. The post-mortem examination of slaughtered animals for religious reasons had given the Jews a knowledge of pathology which the Greeks and others had missed.

Jewish doctors, barred by the Christian Church as infidels, became the secret physicians not only of the well-to-do families but of many monasteries during the Middle Ages. Monks kept them hidden, consulted them about their own ailments.

The biggest contribution which Old Testament medicine made was the Day of Rest: "Six days shalt thou labour and do all thy work . . ."

11. GREEK MEDICINE

According to legend, Aesculapius was the son of Apollo by an earthly maiden and he made Chiron, the centaur, his tutor in the ways of healing. Chiron, the first chirurgeon, taught his pupil well and was surpassed by him.

Pindar, in the third Pythian ode, recounts how Aesculapius became so proficient that he was doing Pluto out of business by diminishing the shades in Hades. Complaint was laid before Zeus, who, always trigger-happy with his thunderbolts, killed Aesculapius and promoted him to Olympus as a god. It must have been an interesting ménage because Apollo, who was already physician-in-ordinary to the Olympians, was also the god whose far-darting arrows, like those of the Second Horseman of the Apocalypse, spread plagues and epidemics, which the Asclepiads, the earthly disciples of his son, were dedicated to preventing.

In this way, mythology gets mixed up with history and we cannot be sure whether Aesculapius was in fact an earthly physician like Imhotep, the Egyptian, who was deified by popular acclaim, as it were. From Homer one would imagine so—that Aesculapius was a flesh-and-blood doctor. He certainly was a fecund one. His daughter Panacea was versed in knowledge of all the earth's remedies and could cure anything (hence "panacea" as a term for an alleged cure-all).

Another daughter, Hygeia, was responsible for public health and social welfare (hence "hygiene"). And her special job around the house was to feed the sacred serpents, which performed healing miracles.

This cult of the serpent was by no means confined to the Greeks. It figures in almost all primitive medicine (including the "snake oil" of the American medical mountebanks). The serpent was synonymous with wisdom. It might know more than was good for it (or us), as in the Garden of Eden, but it knew both good and evil —poison and antidote—and, treated with due respect, was the ally of the doctor. The ancient Greeks, who always had a practical turn of mind, went further: they ate snake meat to make them better doctors.

Telesphorus, who must have been the Peter Pan of Aesculapius's family because he is always represented as a little boy, had the job of ensuring a safe convalescence.

Podalirius, another son, was the specialist in internal medicine and also the father of psychiatry—he diagnosed Ajax's madness by one look at his flashing eyes. He was also a successful physician in a way not unknown in later days. On his way home from the siege of Troy, he was shipwrecked on the coast of Caria. He was taken to the royal palace where the king's daughter was lying mortally ill. Podalirius bled her, saved her life and married her.

Machaon was the surgeon-son, private physician to Menelaus at the siege of Troy. He was one of Homer's heroes, who not only served the wounded nobly but was one of the volunteers for the Wooden Horse. In the midst of battle, when an arrow pierced Menelaus's armor, Machaon rushed to the wounded man, withdrew the shaft, leaving the head to plug the wound, then sucked the wound and applied healing balm. When Machaon himself was wounded by Paris (whose elopement with Helen had brought about the war) Idomeneus cried out to Nestor, passing in his chariot: "Quick, my Lord Nestor, flower of Achaean chivalry! Pick up Machaon in your chariot and drive with all speed to the ships. A surgeon who can cut out an arrow and heal a wound is worth a regiment."

A statistical analysis that has been made of the *Iliad* shows that Homer described 147 war wounds, of which 106 were spear wounds with 80 per cent mortality; 17 sword thrusts with total mortality; 12 arrow wounds with 42 per cent mortality; 12 wounds from slings with 66.7 per cent mortality. The deaths were 77.6 per cent of the total wounded. And, of course, Homeric battle-glory takes no account of unheroic details like dysentery, fevers and the like.

One thing which is clear from the *Iliad* is that by 1000 B.C. medicine was already a highly respected profession. The Asclepieia were temples of the healing cult, and the most celebrated were those of Cos, Epidaurus, Cnidus and Pergamus.

The temples were, in fact, sanatoria with a few priestly trimmings. They were situated on wooded mountains near mineral springs, like modern spas. The patients were received and prepared. The preparation was psychological—a recitation of the achievements of Aesculapius, of the past successes of the temples and their temple remedies. Then there were prayers and sacrifices and the patient was bathed in the mineral springs, followed by oiling and massage. After further ritual, the patient was "incubated," or given temple-sleep. He lay down in the sanctuary and, in the night, a priest in the guise of the god would visit him to administer medical advice if he was awake. If he was asleep and dreamy (and the sleep and dreams may have been medically encouraged) his dreams would later be interpreted or he would be told how the sacred snakes had licked the diseased part and how, if the regimen of drugs or blood-letting or diet were followed, he would be cured. And, of course, if he was not, it would be because he had not enough faith, or had failed in one of the rites, and not because the treatment was at fault; that was, and still is, the excuse of the faith healer. On the other hand, the combination of suggestion and medicine can be efficacious.

The Greeks were the heirs of many cultures. Like the spice trade which was later to converge on Venice, the caravans of knowledge converged on Greece. They were influenced by the Babylonians, the Persians, the Indians, the Egyptians, and by the one great civilization which we have not discussed, the Minoan. In overrunning the Minoan cities of the Levant, including Troy (about 1000 B.C.), the Greeks learned a great deal. The Minoans were particularly advanced in public health, as their excavated drainage systems, water supplies, baths, and refuse-disposal systems show.

Between Aesculapius and Hippocrates—between the Age of Homer and the Age of Pericles—were the philosophers. Medically speaking, philosophy is not very helpful when it *deduces* a system, expects the observed facts to conform and ignores them when they do not. When philosophers, by their intellectual authority, impose a body of doctrine, they can block progress. Pythagoras, of Samos (580-489 B.C.), who set forth the famous theorem: "The area of the square on the hypotenuse of a right-angled triangle is equal to the sum of the area of the squares on the two sides which contain the right angle," may have been a remarkable mathematician, but his doctrine of the mystic medical power of numbers was not much comfort to someone with an ulcer or a toothache. The only thing that can be said of it was that it probably made physicians "number conscious" and was reflected in Hippocrates' useful clinical conception of "critical days."

Anaxagoras of Clazomenae (500-428 B.C.) assumed the four elements—earth, air, fire and water—to be related to everything. This doctrine was spectacularly propounded by Empedocles (504-443 B.C.), who sought to immortalize it and himself (according to the legend, endorsed by the poet, Matthew Arnold) by throwing himself into the crater of Etna:

"To the elements it came from," he says as he poises for the jump,

> "Everything will return—
> Our bodies to earth,
> Our blood to water,
> Heat to fire,
> Breath to air. . . ."

Even if his end was poetic license, it was at least consistent with his theories and his life. According to him and his followers blood was hot; phlegm, cold; black bile moist; and yellow bile dry. Disease was the imbalance of these. To restore health the physician must try to adjust the balance. So, a cold (excessive phlegm) called for a hot remedy. Fever (a surplus of hot blood) called for a cold one. This was the basis of the doctrine of the *humors,* which prevailed in medicine for the next 2000 years.

Empedocles is the classical prototype of the medical mountebank, and his circus act of plunging into the boiling lava of Etna would (true or not) have rejoiced the heart of his American successor, Phineas Barnum. He traveled through the Greek cities, clad in a purple robe, gold-cinctured, long-haired and laurel-crowned, and encouraged people to believe in his supernatural powers. As a self-advertising poet, who did not need any help from Matthew Arnold, he proclaimed his greatness.

"All hail, O friends! but unto ye I walk
As god immortal now, no more as man,
On all sides honoured fittingly and well,
Crowned both with fillets, and with flowering wreaths.
When with my throngs of men and women I come
To thriving cities I am sought by prayers
And thousands follow me. . . ."

Yet, withal, he was a shrewd physician. He checked an epidemic of malarial fever by draining swampy lands. He fumigated houses against infection and improved the health conditions of his native town (Agrigentum in Sicily) by blocking a cleft in a mountainside.

While the physician-philosophers were thus muddling reason with the supernatural, the Greek artists were making a genuine contribution to medical knowledge. This was the age of the Greek athletes, when by exercise they sought, not only to excel in sports, but to remedy any defect in a limb or an organ. With hundreds of nude youths wrestling, jumping, running and throwing, the sculptors of the day had opportunities for observing the anatomical detail of the healthy body. From such masterpieces of anatomical observation as the *Doryophorus* of Praxiteles, the *Apoxyomenos* of Lysippus, the *Nike* of Paionios, and such studies of violent muscular action as the *Borghese Warrior* (Lysippus), the *Farnese Bull* and the *Laocoon* (Rhodian school), one could teach muscular anatomy today.

But the Greeks did not practice human dissection so

they had little knowledge of the internal anatomy of the organs, etc. True, Aristotle (384-322 B.C.) dissected animals and thus founded comparative anatomy, as he founded botany, zoology, embryology and physiology. He was so great an experimental research worker that he deserves his place as one of the greatest biologists of all time. For 2000 years he was regarded as so infallible that his judgments could not be challenged and his misconceptions persisted, to the disadvantage of medical progress. For example, he regarded the heart as the seat of the emotions (as poets still believe), of sensation, and of thought. To him the brain was merely a gland supplying the cold humors to prevent the overheating of the body by the heart-furnace.

12. THE FATHER OF MEDICINE: HIPPOCRATES

Now we come to Hippocrates (460-370 B.C.) who can fairly be regarded as the founder of medicine as we know it today. That is to say, he gave it its scientific spirit, replaced superstition by diagnostic observation and clinical treatment, and gave medicine its ethical ideals. The only instruments of precision he had were his open mind and his keen senses. His shrewd descriptions of diseases are models for doctors even nowadays.

He was born on the island of Cos, the son of a doctor, and he studied in Athens and traveled, practicing the art of medicine, in the various cities of Thrace, Thessaly and Macedonia. Cos is famous for its Temple of Aesculapius, the ruins of which still stand on a wooded hillside. Modern historians doubt whether he was ever a member of the temple cult. If he was, he was one of the great apostates of history because his whole teaching was a renunciation of theology and, indeed, of philosophy, which had replaced observation by doctrine.

Thus, instead of blaming disease on the gods, Hippocrates founded the bedside method. Every patient was an original volume to be studied. In every instance he observed the symptoms and nature of the disease as new facts. There was, of course, cross-reference to experience, but only when the facts had been noticed and without any presumption of the facts. In a way, it was rather like doing a crossword puzzle. He took all the clues, examined them over and over again, and fitted them into the "down" and "across" of the pattern of clinical experience. Previously, among the philosopher-physicians, the clues had had to conform to the pattern and not the pattern the clues.

We have the case book records of Hippocrates, although some might suggest that they were the notes of a school rather than of a single man. If so, the master imposed his personality. There are forty-two clinical cases—almost the only records of the kind for the next 1700 years. They are set down with complete objectivity, modesty, and honesty admitting failures.

"I have written this down deliberately," says Hippocrates, "believing it is valuable to learn of unsuccessful efforts and to know the causes of their failure." Thus 60 per cent of his cases are admitted as fatal, with no excuse or any transfer of blame.

Here is a typical case history of the fourth century B.C.:

"The woman with the quinsy, who lodged with Aristion. Her complaint began in the tongue; voice inarticulate; tongue red and parched.

"*First day*: Shivered, then became heated.

"*Third day*: Rigor, acute fever; reddish, and hard, swelling on both sides of the neck and chest; extremities cold and livid; respiration elevated; drink returned through the nose; she could not swallow; bowel and bladder movements suppressed.

"*Fourth day*: All symptoms worse.

"*Fifth day*: Died."

All these centuries later, a doctor could recognize the symptoms as clearly as though he had stood with Hippocrates at the bedside of "the woman who lodged with Aristion." It is diphtheria. The inflamed throat (quinsy); the paralysis of the palate causing food to come back through the nose; the speech difficulties, and the spread of the septic process into the neck and chest—a not uncommon complication—are all consistent with diphtheria.

In every case, the symptoms are graphically described—like those of "Philescos, who lived by the wall," whose breathing throughout his fever was "like that of a person recollecting himself." This in modern medical literature is "Cheyne-Stokes respiration" (defined in 1846). There is a rhythmic variation in intensity of the breathing and then a cessation for several seconds until the patient "recollects himself" and jerks into breathing again.

Hippocrates insisted on *prognosis,* that is, on predicting the course which the disease will take. Shakespeare knew the *Hippocratic facies,* the prognostic signs of approaching death, for he makes the Hostess (Henry V, Act II, Scene iii) say of the last hours of Falstaff—"e'en at the turning o' the tide"—

"For after I saw him fumble with the sheets, and play with flowers, and smile upon the fingers' end, I knew there was but one way; for his nose was as sharp as a pen . . ."

Although Hippocrates knew the use of many drugs, he believed in (and actually used the phrase) "the healing power of Nature" and was sparing in his prescriptions. His treatment was restrained to fresh air, good diet, mild purgatives, modern bloodletting, barley gruel and barley water, honey-and-water, honey-and-vinegar, massage and baths.

Hippocrates is recalled also for his *Aphorisms:*

"Life is short and Art is long; the Crisis is fleeting, Experiment risky, Decision difficult. Not only must the physician be ready to do his duty, but the patients, the attendants, and the patient's surroundings must conduce to the cure."

"When delirium ends in sleep, it is a good sign."

"If there is painful affection in any part of the body and yet no suffering, there is mental disorder."

"Those naturally very fat are more liable to sudden death than the thin."

"Apoplexy is commonest between the ages of forty and sixty."

"Consumption comes most often to those between eighteen and thirty-five years of age."

And many more which are still sound.

And he is remembered in the *Hippocratic Oath,* the basis of professional ethics, which includes:

"Into whatsoever houses I shall enter I shall enter to help the sick and I will abstain from all intentional wrongdoing and harm, especially from abusing the bodies of man or woman, bond or free.

"And whatsoever I shall see or hear in the course of

my profession, as well as outside my profession in my relations with people, if it be what should not be published, I will never divulge, holding such things as holy secrets."

So in Hippocrates, and the school and tradition which stems from him, we have the first real break from magic and mysticism, and the foundations of Rational Medicine. He was, however, the practitioner not of the Science but the Art of Medicine, relying on experience rather than experiment. He has become the embodiment of the Good Physician, the friend of the patient and the humane expert.

Today, 2500 years later, with all the armory of drugs and the panoply of medical science, there is no substitute for the doctor to whom the patient is not just "Case 2735/Z" on the laboratory file but Betsy Brown, worrying less about her own complaint (the one in the lab records) than about Junior's winter underwear, or whether little Eliza is moping, or whether Ed is shooting crap every night with "the boys." She may be a curious serological specimen to the medical scientist, but to her family doctor she is what "The wife of Delearces, who lay sick on the plain, seized after a grief by an acute fever . . ." was to Hippocrates—an object of compassionate understanding.

13. ROMAN MEDICINE

The emperor of half the world had a stomach-ache. His empire stretched from Hadrian's Wall in barbarous Britain to the Caspian Sea. It embraced the cultures of Greece, Egypt, Troy, Assyria, Babylon, and Sumer. Beyond the Pamirs was an empire even greater in extent, better organized and with the most civilized political system in the world—China under the Han Dynasty.

From all over the vast Roman Empire quacks, or doctors with smatterings of medical lore, had drifted into Rome—the herb-gatherers, the drug peddlers, the salve dealers, army surgeons who had seen service with the legions, Wise Women (sagae), occultists and bath attendants. There were the archiatri, the court physicians.

But Marcus Aurelius (161-180 A.D.) had a stomach-ache for which neither his Stoical philosophy nor his archiatri had a cure. To their great indignation, he sent for a Greek who had been a surgeon to the gladiators and who had built up a fashionable practice as a physician in

Rome before the jealousy of his professional colleagues had driven him into exile, to his native Pergamon, in Asia Minor. Now he was back in Rome and summoned to the presence of the emperor.

And so the last of the great Greeks confronted the last of the great Romans.

No one can accuse Galen of modesty. He was about to effect a cure which he himself described as "really marvelous—the most remarkable diagnosis I have ever made."

The emperor had been campaigning with his legions on the Danube frontier, and on his return to Rome had been taken ill with what the court physicians held to be "a feverish paroxysm"—medical ignorance masquerading as a fashionable complaint. They had treated him with purgatives. Three physicians were in attendance in the sickroom when the interloper arrived. They had taken the imperial pulse and had decided that it was the beginning of an attack of paroxysm. Galen stood mockingly aloof.

"Why do you not also examine our pulse, Galen?" querulously demanded the sick emperor.

"Because, Your Majesty," says Galen in his own account, "two of those gentlemen have already done so, and since they have been traveling with you, are more familiar with your pulse and better able to judge of its present condition."

Impatiently the emperor ordered him to take his pulse.

"Considering the age and constitution of the patient, the pulse rate seemed to me inconsistent with an attack of fever and I insisted that none was to be feared. I said that the stomach was overloaded with nourishment which had been coated with phlegm."

Here, of course, he was invoking the Greek "humors." Phlegm was the "cold" humor.

The emperor was much impressed. Three times he repeated. "That is right. It is exactly as thou sayest; I feel that cold food is disagreeing with me." He then asked Galen what was to be done.

"I answered him frankly that if another than the emperor had been the patient I should, following my custom, have given him wine with pepper. 'With sovereigns like thyself, physicians are in the habit of employing the least drastic remedies, therefore, unfortunately it must suffice to apply wool saturated with warm spikenard upon the abdomen.'"

The emperor, with royal condescension, agreed that the respectful remedy for an imperial stomach would be a purple wool and warm ointment. He sent for an attendant to apply it and dismissed Galen from his presence. As soon as he had gone, however, he sent for a flagon of Sabine wine, spiced it heavily with pepper, and, like the most vulgar of his subjects, "broke his wind."

The skill, and medical diplomacy, of Galen duly impressed the emperor.

"He said that at last he had a physician and a courageous one," says Galen. "He said that he had tried many, not only the covetous but also those greedy of fame and honor and those filled with envy and malice, but that I was the first of the physicians and the only philosopher."

Thereafter the emperor and the empress, Faustina, attended the lectures which Galen gave to the public, claiming that the judgment of the ordinary people was often sounder than that of doctors.

Galen was a braggart, and, unlike Hippocrates, reported only such cases as were successful and redounded to his credit. Nevertheless, he was a remarkable physician. He wrote more than 300 books, of which only 118 survived a fire in his own lifetime. He kept twelve scribes busy recording his anatomical observations, his selective case histories, the drugs he prescribed, and his boasts. His thinking was saddled with the Greek "humors." His anatomy was misleading, because, in spite of his experience with the gladiators, he had the prevailing objection to human dissection and drew his human analogies from studies of animals. His works are full of superstition, but the amount of factual observation and common sense suggests that this was deliberate and that he was corrupting his science to suit the fashions of his time. He was certainly a shrewd psychologist and understood what we would now call psychosomatic medicine—the reaction of mental states on organic illness.

A classic case of this was Galen's cure for the wife of Servius Paulus. She was seriously ill and her physician was treating her for organic disease. Galen cured her by making her laugh. Around the town, he had heard her name associated with that of an actor. As he was feeling her pulse he made conversation about the theater and expressed his admiration of the actor's dancing. Her pulse bounded at the mention of his name—an early anticipation of the lie-detector—and he whispered something to her, which made her laugh. Galen was too shrewd to give away either his secret or hers. So we do not know what it was he whispered, but the patient's laugh was the beginning of a cure, in which no doubt the actor played an active part. It is also recorded that Galen was paid the exorbitant fee of 400 gold pieces for the curing of the wife of the Consul Boethus of melancholia.

Galen, the Greek, stands out as the greatest physician in the history of Rome. As far as clinical medicine is concerned it is a depressing history. The Romans were the heirs to the great cultures they had absorbed, including the medical advances made by the school at Alexandria which had extended the works of the Greeks after Hippocrates. But the Romans made few contributions to the knowledge of the human body and its frailties, or to the treatment of the individual patient.

This was due in part to a combination of two factors—the narrow-minded attitude of the earlier Romans, like Cato the Elder, who despised the conquered Greeks as effete, and to superstition.

The Romans preferred to rely on their domestic deities or on their Sibylline Books. These were the prophetic books preserved in the Temple of Jupiter and consulted on occasions of national danger. When both failed, as in the plague of 292 B.C., they might turn to the Greeks. On that occasion a mission was sent to Epidaurus to the Temple of Aesculapius. On the return of the mission an Aesculapian serpent escaped from the ship as it sailed up the Tiber, landed on an island in the river, and miraculously brought an end to the plague. That island became a hospital island, with its rocks carved into the shape of a ship, with Aesculapian symbols on its "prow." Later it became known as the island of St. Bartholomew, and when Rahere, the court jester of Henry I, founded a hospital in the city of London he called it after this island.

Although so backward in clinical medicine, the Romans made outstanding contributions to public health. They had a well-developed army medical service, which accompanied the legions on their campaigns. They instituted base hospitals throughout the empire and established convalescent camps at strategic points throughout the Roman world. Each cohort of 420 men had at least one doctor with it and a high ranking surgeon supervised each legion, or ten cohorts.

Outstanding features of Roman times were the drainage systems like the Cloaca Maxima, the sewer built in the earliest days of Rome and still part of the system of the modern city. Even the remote Roman settlements, even the frontier posts on Hadrian's Wall, had efficient sanitary systems.

Even more remarkable was the provision of fresh water for drinking and for bathing. By A.D. 110, ten great aqueducts were supplying the capital with 40 million gallons of drinking water daily. The private houses had a service pipe with cisterns and taps. Settling tanks and other purification methods were in general use and the plumbing reached a high degree of excellence. They believed in the medical and social advantages of baths. Some of the baths had marble accommodations for as many as 3000 people. They provided for cold baths (*frigidaria*) and warm baths (*tepidaria* and *calidaria*). They realized the virtues of natural springs and they used central heating by means of piping from hollow chambers under the floor. They knew the benefits of town planning, well-ventilated houses, paved streets, and cremation of the dead. They had ordinances governing pure food.

14. THE END OF THE ANCIENT EMPIRES

But all the preoccupation of the Romans with public health could not, in the absence of scientific knowledge of the diseases against which the measures were directed, avert the medical disasters which destroyed an empire. That destruction had already begun and was in progress when Galen cured the emperor of his stomach-ache.

Rome, like China at the same time, was beset on the boundaries of its empire by virile barbarians. In the second century B.C.—around the time of Marcus Aurelius— a great misfortune came upon the Roman and Chinese Empires simultaneously, one which weakened both to barbarian pressure. This was a pestilence of extraordinary virulence. It raged for eleven years in China and destroyed the social framework. The Han Dynasty fell and disorder reigned in China from which the country did not properly recover until the seventh century A.D., when balance was restored by the Tang Dynasty.

The infection spread through Asia into Europe. It raged through the Roman Empire from A.D. 164 to 180. It decimated the garrisons and populations of the Roman provinces. Rulers and ruled were alike afflicted. Administration, like administrators, sickened and collapsed. This pestilence was a disease of the civilized world from which the barbarian races appeared to be immune. The frontiers of both empires became vulnerable, the nomads of the Asian steppes pressed southwards and westwards. The Goths, coming originally from Sweden, had migrated to the Volga region of Russia and to the shores of the Black Sea and had taken ships upon the warm waters and harried the Mediterranean shores. They in turn had felt the pressure of the Huns, coming out of Asia.

And so the Goths and the Visigoths pressed westwards to destroy the Roman Empire. Their advance guards, their flying columns, their panzers, had been the invisible armies of disease.

Ironically, because Galen was so industrious in his writings and so often right in his facts, and because he was so confident and dogmatically arrogant in his knowledge, he—who might have advanced medical inquiry—braked it. Galen, as far as the pontiffs and pundits of the Dark Ages were concerned, had said everything. Even as late as 1559, the College of Physicians in London condemned one of its fellows, Dr. John Geynes, and forced him to recant, when he dared to suggest that Galen's works contained errors.

Galen's authority, during the next thousand years, was due to the fact that in philosophy he was a monotheist, believing in one God, and so his medical teachings were acceptable to the religions of both Christendom and Islam.

So, when Galen was called to the palace to treat the imperial stomach-ache, it was to the sickbed not only of an emperor but of an empire.

Western civilization was about to enter upon a thousand years of darkness. And Galen, the bright moon of Roman medicine, was himself to pass across the face of the sun in that eclipse.

Part Three

A THOUSAND YEARS
OF DARKNESS

> With us ther was a DOCTOUR OF
>   PHISIK
> In all this world ne was ther noon hym
>   lik
> To speke of phisik and of surgerye;
> For he was grounded in astronomye.
> He kepte his pacient a ful greet deel
> In houres by his magyk natureel.
> Wel koude he fortunen the ascendent
> Of his ymages for his pacient.
> He knew the cause of everich maladye,
> Were it of hoot, or cold, or moyste or
>   drye,
> And where they engendred and of what
>   humour.

—CHAUCER: Prologue, *Canterbury Tales*

1. DOCTOUR OF PHISIK

When April with its sweet showers had pierced the drought of March to the roots, Chaucer assembled his pilgrims at the Tabard Inn in Southwark, on the south bank of the Thames. Thirty, including Chaucer, were to set out for Canterbury. There is a doubt about the exact year, but it was somewhere about 1385. Such pilgrimages had become a fashion since the Black Death, when the survivors had journeyed to the shrine of St. Thomas to give thanksgiving for their deliverance.

Like the great plague which in Galen's time had undermined the Roman Empire, the Black Death came out of Asia. It was brought to Messina from the Near East by a Genoese ship in 1347. People fleeing from its horrors took the disease with them, spread it first all over Sicily; then into Tuscany; and then all over Europe. Even Greenland did not escape. Eric the Red had first migrated from Iceland to Greenland in the tenth century and the Norse-

72

men had kept in touch—a contact which was to be fatal, because it seemed that the entire community of Iceland was wiped out. So disease deflected history, because these Greenland Norsemen were, as we know now, already questing down the coast of the American continent and knew the route there at least 150 years before Columbus. The Black Death broke this bridge between the Old World and the New.

The devastations of the Black Death were appalling. Some estimates put deaths at half the entire population of Europe, during the period 1348-59. According to Guy de Chauliac three-quarters of the people of France died. It is said that in London scarcely one in ten survived. Boccaccio, whose Decameron was written around the fugitives from the plague, reported that in Florence, out of 130,000, more than 100,000 died. In that plague, the doctors, or what passed for doctors, could do nothing.

That is not quite true. They could collect their fees, like Chaucer's Doctour of Phisik, who "kepte that he wan in pestilence"—kept what he earned in the pestilence. The description of this medical gentleman is a thumbnail sketch of the state of medicine in the Middle Ages. He was a "big shot" for, in addition to knowing about physic and surgery, he was "grounded in astronomye" (by which Chaucer means "astrology"). We are told that he always attended his patient carefully at times of planetary conjunctions so as to treat at the right moment. He watched for a favorable star, or a sign of the zodiac, which would be fortunate for his patient. He knew the cause for every malady, whether it was hot or cold, or moist or dry, and where it arose and of what humor.

So here we have the physician prescribing according to superstition for sicknesses which depended on the humors or temperament of his patient. His patient was compounded of four elements; blood (fire), phlegm (earth), black bile (water) and yellow bile (air). He could tell at a glance the temperament of his patient. A sanguine fellow "inclining to be fat and prone to laughter" had more than his ration of hot, moist blood. A phlegmatic person would be thickset and slow and lazy because he had too much cold phlegm. The choleric person, having hot yellow bile, would be quick to anger, for little reason. The melancholy man, having too much cold, dry black bile would be pensive, peevish, and fond of his own company.

This theory of the humors and the body fluids dominated medical thinking until the mid-nineteenth century when Virchow published his *Cellular Pathology*. In it he explained the cells which make up the body tissue, and which in some instances (i.e., that of the glands) themselves generate the chemicals which affect our "temperament."

The Medical Pilgrim was well read.

> Wel knew he the olde Esculapius
> And Deyscorides and eek Rufus,
> Olde Ypocras, Haly and Galyen,
> Serapion, Razis and Avycen,
> Avverois, Damascien and Constantyn,
> Bernard and Gatesden and Gilbertyn.

"Esculapius," "Galyen" (Galen), "Ypocras" (Hippocrates) and "Deyscorides" (Dioscorides) we have already met, but who were his other authorities?

2. *RED-BEARD OF EPHESUS*

Rufus, the red-bearded Ephesian who lived in the time of Trajan (A.D. 98-117) made real contributions to medicine. He made a study of the eye, described the crystalline lens, the membranes and hollow center. He made shrewd observations of the pulse and the heartbeats, studied skin diseases and produced a treatise on bubonic plague. His prescriptions were sensible and his surgery competent. He knew, for instance, how to stanch blood by constricting the arteries, by tying the blood vessels, by cautery and by employing astringents (like the styptics a barber uses to stanch a razor cut). He bamboozled later thinking by his wrong description of the liver—having confused pig's liver with the human organ. But, most probably, the Doctour of Phisik, being a fashionable physician, knew him from his treatise on gout, which had been translated into dog-Latin in the sixth century.

3. *HALI, THE MAGI*

Hali ben Abbas, who died in 994, was a Persian magus. He wrote *Almaleki* (The Royal Book), which became a sort of medical bible of Arab, or Moslem, doctors. It was translated into Latin by Stephen of Antioch in the century before Chaucer and had become the textbook of the College of Salerno (of which more anon). It gives a fair account of smallpox and "Persian Fire" (malignant anthrax) and a crude anatomical description of the body.

4. SERAPION, JUNIOR

There were three *Serapions* who were Arab physicians. This was probably one of the sons, who was a slick dispenser and had compiled a list of drugs which the Medical Pilgrim would no doubt have found handy. He obviously did not know a much better pharmacological source—the Persian, Abu Mansur, who compiled (about A.D. 970) a collection of 585 drugs, of which 466 were vegetable, 75 mineral and 44 animal.

5. PRINCE OF PHYSICIANS

Avycen was *Ibn Sina* (A.D. 980-1037), a rollicking character. He was a Persian who wandered round the courts of the Eastern Caliphate as well-regarded by men (and especially women) as a boon companion as he was as the Prince of Physicians. At ten he knew the Koran by heart. At seventeen he knew all that was to be known about philosophy, natural history, poetry, mathematics, law and medicine. At eighteen, he cured a potentate and rummaged the royal archives for further knowledge. At Hammadan, he cured the reigning prince of colic and was made prime minister. His abuse of this office made the people threaten revolt and the emir banished him—only to call him back to cure another bout of colic. He became chief physician of Baghdad's celebrated hospital and wrote a million words on medicine, in intervals between feasting and philandering.

Although he must obviously have been a shrewd doctor, his writings—immensely popular about the time of Chaucer—were part of the bumblings which bedeviled progress. He set men arguing why breasts did not grow on the stomach, why the stomach was not where the brain is, and why the calves are on the back of the legs instead of the front. He discussed the nature of love and decided that it was a mental disease. With Galen, he dominated medical thinking throughout the Middle Ages—until Paracelsus, in 1527, publicly burned the works of both of them.

6. RHASES, THE LUTE-PLAYER

Razis, or *Rhases* (A.D. 860-932) was born in Basra and until he was too old to be the matinee idol of the harems of Baghdad, played the lute and told stories. Then he discovered an interest in medicine. With his lute (and tablets on which to take notes from the Wise Women and the herbalists), he went to Jerusalem, to Cairo, and wandered through North Africa to Spain, where Arab medicine, in the wake of the Saracens, had established the hospitals and academies of Cordova. That was a city of a million people and (reputedly) a thousand baths, with street lighting and elementary schools for children. He learned from the alchemists as he had learned from the Wise Women. He became an intern and studied cases at the bedside, as Hippocrates had done. And he became one of the great clinicians.

On his return to Baghdad, he was ordered by the Caliph to build a new hospital. He hung up pieces of fresh meat in various parts of the city and, more than a thousand years before Pasteur, chose the site where the meat putrefied most slowly (because the atmosphere was purer).

7. AVERROES, THE COMMENTATOR

Avverois, or *Averroes,* was a Moorish physician, born in Cordova in 1126. He was the pupil of another great doctor of the Western Caliphate (Arab Spain), Avenzoar, who dared to dispute the infallibility of Galen and gave his students free-ranging observant minds.

What makes his appearance in the *Canterbury Tales* surprising is the fact that he was anathematized by the medieval Church and had been persecuted in his own lifetime because he was a freethinker whose writings implied a denial of Creation and of personal immortality. On the other hand, his work was profoundly influenced by the Jews, who in their wanderings had found a respite from persecution in Moslem Spain. This combination of Jew and Arab in a Semitic culture was important in medicine. While the Arabs were deficient in anatomical knowledge, the Jews had important insight. The Talmudic practices, to discover what was *kosher* and *terephah*, which required post-mortem examinations of slaughtered animals, had provided knowledge of the characteristics of organic disease.

8. THE DAMASCENE

Damascien was another Arab philosopher-physician. He belonged to the ninth century and to Damascus, also an important medical center in the Arab world. It boasted a great hospital and one of the earliest examples of "socialized medicine." While, of course, the Koran enjoins that the good Moslem must give alms to the poor, this was comprehensive medicine, free to rich and poor alike.

Ibn Al-Alhir gives a description of how he was taken ill on a journey from Jerusalem: "I rode into Damascus to find a physician and was directed to the great hospital. The director greeted me and asked me, in kindly fashion, the nature of my illness. I told him and he wrote me down a prescription and said: 'The attendant will bring you what I have written.' I protested that, by grace of Allah, I was rich enough to pay for my drugs, without depriving the poor, thus, of what they might have. He replied, 'Excellency, you may deny yourself our medicines but do not despise our benefits. In Allah's name, I assure you that the Sultan and his sons and their whole families send here for treatment and cannot pay.' I still protested and said that I could not approve. 'So be it,' he said, 'but it is our duty to minister to all believers, rich or poor, without reckoning.' "

Other accounts tell of wayfarers arriving at the great hospital of Damascus, being only tired in body or in spirit, and being given the comforts that were available for all—young chicken and sherbet and sweetmeats. But after three days they were prescribed an unpleasant medicine—as a hint that they had outstayed their welcome.

9. CONSTANTINE, THE AFRICAN

Constantine, like St. Augustine (not the St. Augustine who was the first Archbishop of Canterbury but he of the *Confessions* and *The City of God*), was born in North

Africa (A.D. 1020). He became a student of oriental languages and wandered in the Middle East, learning the cults and philosophies, including medicine. When he returned to his native Carthage, he was regarded as a magician and persecuted. He fled to Italy and found his way to Salerno, the first medical college of Christendom, and ended his days as a monk in the monastery of Monte Cassino.

He was probably more of a linguist and a translator than a practitioner of medicine, for he knew Arabic, Hebrew and Greek and so collated knowledge into Latin. What, in fact, he did was to make the "heretical" knowledge of Moslem and Jew acceptable in the tongue of Christendom. He produced a lot of mutilated thinking because much of the Arab works which he paraphrased were themselves Moslem paraphrases of the works of Hippocrates and Galen, as received, at second-hand, from the Greek Nestorian Christians who had sought refuge in Persia, A.D. 489.

10. GILBERT, THE ENGLISHMAN

"*Gilbertyn*" died in 1250. He was an Englishman and the leading exponent of Anglo-Norman medicine. He was a sensible fellow who favored the simple treatments and methods of Hippocrates but candidly admitted that he would have seemed an "odd fish" if he had employed them. So he subscribed to a lot of the nonsense and superstition of his time. Here, for instance, is Gilbert's ointment for gout:

"Take a very fat puppy and skin him. Then take the juice of wild cucumber, rue, pellitory, ivy berries, juniper berries, euphorbium, castoreum, fat of vulture, goose, fox and bear, in equal parts, and stuff the puppy therewith. Then boil him. Add wax to the grease which floats to the top and apply as an ointment. Or, if you prefer, take a frog when neither sun nor moon is shining, cut off its hind legs and wrap them in deerskin. Apply the frog's right leg to the right foot and the left leg to the left foot of the gouty patient and for certain he will be cured."

He also produced a weird and wonderful hygiene guide for great overlords and their ladies when they made court progresses by land or sea.

Gilbert's serious contributions were an original account

of leprosy which became the basis of medieval ordinances, and his recognition that smallpox was a contagious disease.

11. BERNARD, THE SCOTSMAN

Bernard de Gordon, a Scotsman, was a teacher from 1285 to 1307 at the medical school of Montpellier, founded A.D. 738. His book *The Lily of Medicine* is a typical exercise of the time—that bleak, thought-ingrowing age—full of subtle, meaningless reasoning, superstition, dogma and borrowed experience.

It is notable for one thing—the first reference to the use of spectacles. He calls them *oculus berellinus*—an "eye" made from a "smoky stone." (Berill? Beryl? One pauses, because beryllium, now so important as a mineral of the Atomic Age, is akin to emerald, and Pliny refers to Nero's watching the gladiators in the Coliseum through an emerald lens.) Of course, Roger Bacon had proposed, in a book sent to the pope in 1267, that a segment of a glass sphere should be used as a reading glass by elderly people.

12. THE DOCTOUR HIMSELF

And, lastly, *John of Gaddesden* (A.D. 1280-1361). He was a prebendary of St. Paul's, physician to King Edward II, and a professor of Merton College, Oxford. His medical treatise *English Rose,* compiled in 1314, is a shoddy affair. It shows him to be a creature full of superstition, uncritically purveying quack medicines, avaricious and a grubber, not of the virtues of hedgerow medicine, but of the garbage heap.

But before he is utterly discarded we should remember that when Edward II's son had smallpox, he reduced the pitting and disfigurement by hanging red cloth round the patient. No doubt it was on a par with the rest of his superstitious lore, compounded with conventional Galenism and the humors. Red was a mystical color as much resented by demons as by Spanish bulls. It was also identified with the flush of fever, so it was "like treating like" —just as my great-grandmother believed when she wrapped a red flannel scarf around an inflamed throat. Moreover, red light was supposed to draw out the "choler" of a fever by attracting the blood to the surface of the skin where it could be cooled.

All these things probably influenced the pixilated Royal Physician but, by applying the red cloth, he was, no doubt, quite unconsciously practicing "phototherapy." Over 500 years later, in 1893, Finsen, the pioneer of light-treatment, showed that the pustules of smallpox could be reduced by the exclusion of ultraviolet light, just as lupus, the tuberculous skin disease, could be helped by concentrations of ultraviolet rays. Red curtains would serve the same purpose.

John of Gaddesden, that "verray parfit praktisour," could "cure" epileptic fits with a necklace, and palsy with aqua vitae, and, according to Freind, who wrote the *History of Physick,* he "is very artful in laying baits for the Delicate, for the Ladies, for the Rich. He condescends to instruct them even in Perfumes and washes; especially how to dye their hair. And such is his respect for the Rich that he is always studying to invent some of the most select and dearest medicine for them; and of these is a very good thing indede, for he orders twice the quantity for them as he does for the poor."

John of Gaddesden was Chaucer's contemporary and, according to some authorities, was the model for the Medical Pilgrim—with the reference to "Gatesden" deliberately intended to disguise a character too powerful to offend with quips like:

> For gold in phisick is a cordial
> Therefore he lovede gold in special.

13. SICKNESS SANCTIFIED

With the collapse of the Roman Empire, the Church had become the repository of knowledge—of those facts, not only of medicine but of learning generally, which had drained through thousands of years into the Mediterranean: From Aryan-Dravidian India, from Persia, Sumer, Assyria, Babylon, Minoa, Egypt and Greece and across the Spice Road from China and the Orient. That knowledge had been enthroned by Alexander in Alexandria. There Ptolemy, the geographer, Euclid, Archimedes, Hero, Dioscorides, Soranus, Galen, Hierophilus, Erasistratus (who used the water clock to time the pulse) and many others had studied, and endowed its great libraries and museums. In 391, in the Christian riots in Alexandria, the destruction of temples included that of Jupiter Serapis and with it the remains of a library which had once totaled 700,000 rolls of manuscripts.

Such medical knowledge as survived was scattered through the monasteries and dispersed among the many Orders of the Church. And for eight centuries research stood still. Hippocrates had taught that illness was not a punishment sent by the gods but something to be studied as other natural phenomena were studied. Now, under the Church, the older views of the supernatural origins of disease were revived.

St. Augustine, in the fifth century, had said: "All diseases of Christians are to be ascribed to demons, chiefly do they torment the fresh baptized; yea, even the guiltless, new-born infant."

So, since disease implied demonic possession, the sick were treated by the monks through prayers, laying on of hands, exorcism, penances, and the exhibition of holy relics. No doubt it worked. Apart from psychogenic and hysteric illness which will respond to faith cures, most illnesses, except when death occurs, cure themselves— in time and with suffering. And every cure redounded to the glory of the Church.

Some monks were more enterprising and discovered that there was a profitable traffic in more mundane treatments, and so bishops and abbots and abbesses substituted for a medical profession. Armed with a smattering of Galen; a borrowing from the cabalists; a seasoning of alchemy from Islam; a recourse to the Jewish physicians, whom many monasteries kept hidden; and a few incantations and magical amulets and charms, they treated the sick. The extent of such practices was so great that Pope Innocent III, in 1139, barred priests from the dispensing of medicine. But they persisted. Thirty years later Pope Alexander III threatened churchmen who attended medical lectures with excommunication. St. Bernard, founder of the Cistercian Order, not only forbade his monks from studying or practicing medicine but from having any recourse to treatment for their own ailments. "To buy drugs, to consult physicians, or to take medicines befits not religion," was his ordinance.

More serious, in its way, was the Edict of Tours, in 1163. This declared that the Church abhorred the shedding of blood (not, of course, in wars) and made surgery, and through it the better knowledge of the human body, a disreputable practice.

Then there was the Bull of Pope Boniface VII (1300) which was to cripple anatomical research even more. It decreed that whoever dared to cut up a human body or boil it would fall under the ban of the Church. In fact, the decree was not directed against the anatomists at all. It was aimed at the Crusaders, who, in order to ship home the remains of their dead for burial in ancestral tombs, had, to the scandal of the Church, cut up and boiled the bodies to obtain the skeletons for easy shipment. But the decree was applied as a ban on dissection and post-mortem examination.

Textbooks illustrated with diagrams showing how the various parts of the body had affinities with the signs of the zodiac now had to be cleansed of such pagan symbolism. Zodiacal signs were replaced by the names of saints. St. Bernadine was identified with the lungs; St. Appollonea with the teeth; St. Lawrence with the back; St. Blaise with the throat; St. Agatha with the breasts; St. Erasmus with the abdomen; and St. Just with the head. And diseases, too, were put under the special jurisdiction of particular saints. Chorea still remains "St. Vitus Dance." Ergotism is "St. Anthony's Fire." St. Valentine was concerned with epilepsy.

14. LANTERNS IN THE DARK

So, in general, it was the Dark Ages. That is, if we are thinking only of the learning and medicine of the West.

In the East, this was the age of *Susruta* and the *Vagbhata,* the Hindu advances in surgery and medicine, and of the great volumes of Chinese medicine. Keh Hung (A.D. 281-360) in the Tsin Dynasty published his *Handbook of Emergencies*. The Tang Dynasty (618-906) sponsored the great encyclopedias, and in the Sung Dynasty paper books spread the knowledge of particular diseases. In Arab medicine, there were progressive minds and institutions.

There were a few bright gleams even in the West— like the founding of the College of Salerno in Italy. The beaches of Salerno were to have a headline significance as a battlefield in the Second World War but in the fourth century Salerno was a salubrious, peaceful spot, which was chosen as the site of the first medical school in Christendom. The Church had no part in its foundation. Reputedly it was started by four masters: Elinus, the Jew; Pontus, the Greek; Adale, the Arab; and Salernus, the Latin.

Nearby was the monastery of Monte Cassino, founded by St. Benedict in 529. There was a friendly relationship between the medical school and the monastery, and the school itself was lay and liberal, and open to students of all languages and nationalities. Arab and Jewish physicians taught there and women were admitted to the faculty.

During the Crusades, Monte Cassino was a kind of base hospital to which Crusaders were brought from the Holy Land, and when the Normans took over Sicily they encouraged the exchange of learning. In 1140, Roger II of Sicily instituted the first medical degree with the following ordinance: "Whosoever shall henceforth practice medicine, let him present himself to our officials and judges and be examined by them." Dire penalties were threatened to quacks who dared practice without qualifying.

Salerno also laid down a code of medical ethics and professional conduct, including: "Look not desirously on the man's wife, daughter or handmaid, for this blinds the eyes of the physician, deprives him of divine assistance and disturbs the patient's mind." There is much sly medical advice also: "When you feel the pulse remember that it may be affected by your arrival, or, the patient being mean, by his thinking about your fee. . . ."

Among the wounded Crusaders succored at Salerno was Robert, Duke of Normandy, son of William the Conqueror, who dallied so long that he lost his throne. One of his diversions at Salerno is alleged to have been the supervision of a handbook of medicine, written in Latin doggerel but full of sensible advice, which both humanized and humorized medicine when, later, it had a wide currency.

The three physicians recommended as best in the textbook of Salerno were "First, Doctor *Quiet,* next Doctor *Merry-Man,* then Doctor *Diet.*"

Salerno had a healthy influence (in all senses of the term) and, although its supremacy was later disputed by the schools of Montpellier, Bologna, Paris and Padua, it remained a center of medical learning until closed by Napoleon.

15. PLAGUES AND PESTILENCE

Although deficient in medical knowledge, the Dark Ages were not entirely lacking in the Christian virtue of charity towards the sick poor, and hospitals and lazarhouses were fairly general. Having in mind, however, the appallingly unsanitary conditions of the cities, where all the lessons of such things as drainage, which had been known since 3000 B.C., had been forgotten, one wonders whether the hospitals were not themselves rather the pesthouses of infection.

Anyway, it was a civilization (?) ill-equipped to withstand the horrors of the Black Death. Such doctors as there were could do nothing against the plague, and the people, brought up on superstitions, were overwhelmed by the holocaust of infection. God and all the saints had deserted them.

Thus we have the grotesque, macabre manifestations of mass hysteria like the Dancing Mania, the Flagellants, and the insensate pogroms of the Jews.

The most severe outbreak of Dancing Mania occurred first at Aix-la-Chapelle in 1374, after a recurrence of the Black Death. It spread through the Netherlands and western Germany. Men and women and children lost all control, joined hands and danced in a frenzy in the streets for hours until they fell in their tracks. They shrieked, saw visions, and maimed one another. Modern authorities think that this may have been due, in the first instance, to a virus which attacked the nervous system and that there must have been organic disease in many cases, because there are frequent references to abdominal swellings and pain which made the dancers bind their stomachs with bandages. But it is also plain that the hysteria itself was infectious and that people who watched lost mental and emotional control and rocked and rolled.

The Flagellants, a cult formed in the latter part of the thirteenth century, were a strange brotherhood who went from town to town slashing one another with whips until their bare backs streamed with blood. In the wake of the Black Death the cult spread to the ordinary people, lashing insanely to beat out the demons of diseases for which superstitious medicine offered neither cure nor comfort.

These mass afflictions of disease were yet another pretext for the persecution of the Jews, who were accused of causing the plague by poisoning the wells. Lynch law took over. All over western Europe, Jews were seized upon as the scapegoats. In Narbonne, Carcassonne and Burgundy, fifty thousand Jews were burned.

Rats, lice and filth disfigured medieval Europe, which was bankrupt not only in knowledge of how to treat individual patients but also of elementary hygiene. Epidemic followed epidemic—Black Death; sweating sickness (probably a form of influenza); mass ergotism, due to the fungus on the blighted rye of the bread of the poor; St. Vitus Dance and Dancing Mania; venereal disease; leprosy and more plague.

It is a dismal story from which it is a relief to escape into "The Age of the Eye" and to trace the new discoveries which were eventually to add up to the medical science of our own times.

Part Four

THE GREAT ADVANCES (I)

> Medicine is not merely a science but an art. It does not consist in compounding pills, and plasters and drugs of all kinds, but it deals with the processes of life which must be understood before they can be guided. A powerful will may cure when doubt would end in failure. The character of the physician may act more powerfully upon the patient than all the drugs employed.
>
> —PARACELSUS (1490-1541)

1. THE AGE OF THE EYE

Refugees were fleeing westwards. Constantinople had fallen to the Turks in 1453. The Byzantine Empire had come to an end and its scholars had scattered. Not for the last time in the tortured history of mankind were Displaced Persons to repay those who gave them sanctuary by infusing new knowledge and revitalizing their cultures. These fugitives brought with them the Renaissance, by which is meant the rebirth of learning, but "learning" in the sense of acquiring and advancing knowledge and not just of brooding over it as the Schoolmen of the preceding centuries had done. They had made the mind a beleaguered citadel, resisting the facts of the world around them. *Thinking,* to them, had been *believing.*

But the Renaissance might well be called *The Age of the Eye.* For *seeing* became *believing.* Observation replaced speculation. As Ambroise Paré (1510-90) rumbled in his quarrel with Gourmelen, the professor of medicine, in Paris;

"Dare you teach me surgery? You, who have never come out of your study! Surgery is learned by the eye and the hand. You, my little master, know only how to chatter in a chair."

Nor was it merely by accident that the artists contributed so much to the advance of medicine at this time.

They turned the inward eye of learning outwards, seeing the human body as it really was and not as a passage in Aristotle or Galen. Michelangelo, Raphael and Dürer, in the cause of art, minutely studied the human body. Dürer, when he wanted to consult his doctor about a complaint, sent him a nude self-portrait, showing the location of his pain exactly in the region of the spleen. Titian, or, at least, his school, illustrated the remarkable anatomical works of Vesalius. And, ranking with the greatest of his medical contemporaries and, indeed, with the anatomists of any age, was that universal genius, Leonardo da Vinci.

2. THE VERSATILE GENIUS

"Genius" is an overworked and devalued word, but, no matter what measurements or criteria we apply, da Vinci qualified for this description.

One takes a deep breath before reciting the fields in which he excelled—a giant in each: painter of the *Last Supper* and the *Mona Lisa* or *La Gioconda;* sculptor; mathematician; palaeontologist, who used the evidence of the fossils to challenge the dating of the Flood; cosmologist, who proclaimed "The Sun does not move" at a time when such an utterance could have meant the stake; aerodynamist, who conceived the first helicopter; naval architect, who designed the first submarine; military engineer, who invented a breech-loading gun; mechanical engineer, who designed a power-driven spinning mill and a rotary lathe; geologist, physicist and chemist. . . .

It is necessary to draw a second breath to recount his out-of-his-time transcendence as an anatomist. By candlelight, the versatile genius carried out dissection, when it was anathematized by the Church, on over thirty bodies in the Santo Spirito mortuary at Rome. From these dissections he produced about a thousand drawings. Ignoring the writings of the misleading authorities, he started with the body as his textbook. He injected wax into the organs before dissecting them.

He studied the anatomy of the heart, the lungs and the womb. He paid special attention to the valves in the blood vessels and carried out experiments which showed that they operated so that the blood would always flow one way and not be able to reverse back into the heart. He missed the fact that the blood did not percolate from one side of the heart to the other (as Galen had insisted) and so failed to anticipate the discovery of the complete circulation of the blood which Harvey was to make a century later. He was the first to study fully the fetal membranes and the cerebral nerves. He dissected the brain and noted the muscles and their functions. When he decided to study the eye, he boiled it in white of egg and cut it into solidified cross-sections.

Nor did he confine his researches to the dead body. No artist has so carefully depicted the range of human emotions—the fear of the man on the gallows; the anguish of the man in pain; the expression of the man with goiter and the changing physiognomy of age. When he wanted to study the action of the muscles, he constructed wire cages round the limbs. He used optical glasses for magnification, years before Janssen invented the microscope.

If it had not been that Marco Antonio della Torre, with whom he was projecting an encyclopedia on anatomy, died, Leonardo would have preceded Vesalius as "The Father of Anatomy." As it was, his anatomical drawings were lost sight of for nearly 200 years.

3. THE FATHER OF ANATOMY

Some would say that modern medicine began with Andreas Vesalius in 1543. That was the date of the first comprehensive textbook of human anatomy—*De Humani Corporis Fabrica*. It belongs to the perpetual archives of mankind, as the A B C of a new science and as a new experience in art. The text is impressive but the drawings are not less remarkable. Some have been attributed to Titian, and many to Titian's pupil Stephen van Calcar.

Vesalius (1514-64) was born in Brussels, but his family had come from Wesel (hence "Vesalius"). He first studied medicine at Louvain and then went to Paris—to be angered by the Galenic professors who were teaching medicine as an academic exercise. In protest, Vesalius and some of his fellow students defied the teachers and the Church, and set out to study the human body they were supposed to be treating.

Those were the days of hanging and drawing and quartering, of torture, and of burning which made scruples about dissection a quaint deceit. There was no shortage of bodies. Gibbets were plentiful by the wayside and there was a forest of gallows at Montfaucon. There, with macabre enjoyment, François Villon and the student-vagabonds of Paris had picnicked by moonlight until Villon himself was threatened with the fate of his fellow cutthroats and cutpurses.

In this Golgotha, Vesalius and his friends stole corpses and skeletons from the vultures and studied them until, blindfold, they could identify any bone of the skeleton by touch, and, with this knowledge, outraged their professors by contradicting them and the ideas of Galen.

In 1537, Vesalius became professor of anatomy at Padua. Notice that he was only twenty-three years of age and yet occupied a chair at what was then a leading medical school of Europe. His lively lectures attracted as many as 500 students at a session, for his reputation drew them from all over the Continent. To them, he added visual aids—charts of the muscles, skeleton, blood system and generative organs. It was as revolutionary as broadcasting an operation on television.

As Sir Michael Foster wrote: "Five years he wrought, not weaving a web or fancied thoughts, but patiently disentangling the pattern of the texture of the human body, trusting to no word and to no master, admitting nothing except that which he himself had seen. . . ." At the age of twenty-eight he had unveiled the body.

Then the purblind fury of the academic world burst upon him. The teaching centers of the whole of Europe were in a ferment. Jacobus Sylvius, who had been his teacher, denounced Vesalius as a charlatan. His students, in this brimstone atmosphere of medieval McCarthyism, renounced him and denounced him lest they themselves should be smeared. The ecclesiastics reached for the torch to fire the fagots of the man who had defied the Church, had tampered with the human body, and questioned authorities whom religion had accepted. Vesalius, unlike his fellow student Servetus, was not of the stuff of martyrs. Servetus had shown that, in truth, the blood moved from the heart to the lungs, "where it is made red," and had included this unorthodoxy in a tract of Christianity. His "heresies" caused him to fly from Catholic France to Calvinist Geneva, where the Reformers, no less ruthlessly indignant, burned him, and his book, at the stake.

Vesalius was more discreet. He quietly left Padua and secured for himself adequate protection as the court physician of Charles V, but his position became less secure with the succession of the bigoted Philip II, and, as a double insurance, he went off on a pilgrimage to the Holy Land. On his way back, he was shipwrecked on the island of Zante and died of starvation and exposure at the age of fifty. But he had established the "fabric" of the human body.

4. BOMBAST

There was nothing of the courtier or the temporizer about Theophrastus Bombastus von Hohenheim (1490-1541). A bombast, both by name and by nature, he flouted authority and offended his origins. He was the son of a Swiss nobleman but his companions for most of his life were the commonest of common people—public executioners, barbers, gypsies, miners, brothelkeepers, and strolling players. He was the Sir John Falstaff of medicine. But he is secure among the immortals as Philippus Aureolus Paracelsus.

He called himself "Paracelsus"—"beyond Celsus"— boasting an affinity with one of the few classical authorities whom he respected. Celsus, who lived in the reign of Tiberius Caesar, completed in A.D. 30 a monumental work on medicine, full of sound sense, with practical instructions in surgery which would serve even today, and shrewd descriptions of diseases and procedures for treatment. Yet he was not, apparently, a physician, but a Roman patrician concerning himself with the care and treatment of his dependents. His Latinic simplicity contrasted with the bombastic style of Bombastus, who borrowed his name.

Because of his behavior, Paracelsus is liable to be dismissed as a mountebank. Rather he should be accepted as a peacock in a field of crows. In a drab, musty world of Schoolmen he was a flamboyant rebel. He jeered at their pedantry and pomposity, flouted their authority and rejected their authorities. At a time when heretics and their works were being burned, this "heretic," when he was appointed professor of medicine at Basel, took the hallowed works of Galen and Avicena and burned them in the public square. And he broke all traditions of the academics by lecturing in German, instead of Latin, and out of his own experience instead of out of books.

As Sir William Osler said: "Paracelsus was the Luther of medicine, for when authority was paramount he stood out for independent study."

He had had the advantage of his father's fine library, and, as a youngster, had dabbled in occult mysteries of which he never got quit, but here again it is fair to ask whether his "arcana" (mysteries) and astrological extravagances, his gnomes and salamanders, were not part of his showmanship; his compromise with the current superstitions in order to propagate the practical values of his observant medicine. He was a public relations officer out of his time.

He qualified as a doctor of medicine at Ferrara and wandered over the then known world—even, it is suggested, in the Far East, where he may have learned about the metallic drugs and picked up theosophic lore.

Apart from his contemporary eminence as a physician he has a permanent place as the founder of modern chemistry and pharmacy. Alchemy, according to Paracelsus, was "neither to make gold nor silver but to make the supreme sciences and to direct them against disease."

5. ARMY BARBER

"I dressed the wounds and God healed them." That may seem a proper and pious sentiment from one who had learned his craft as a barber's apprentice, who had no formal education, and had acquired all he knew about surgery on the battlefields. But the humility of Ambroise Paré (1510-90) was something more than simple piety; it was the embodiment of a truth which is only now being redeemed in twentieth-century medicine; it was, as he demonstrated in his own practices, a recognition of the Whole Man in the process of healing. We may give it fancy names—call it "psychosomatic medicine"—but it still remains what Paré discovered: the interplay of body and mind.

Perhaps this interplay is best exemplified by Paré's own treatment of the Marquis d'Aurel. At the end of a long professional life, with thirty years spent on the field of war and in the service of four monarchs, he had retired when he was asked by the king to go to the help of a young marquis tortured for seven months, almost to the point of death, by a gunshot wound which had shattered his thigh. Paré took one look at the patient and regretted that he had taken on the case.

"I found him in high fever, his eyes sunk into his head, with a yellowish face, his tongue dry and parched and his body wasting away, and his voice was husky like that of a man near death."

Here is the portrait of a patient poisoned by the sepsis of an infected and neglected wound. The marquis was lying in appalling filth because his medical attendants had not dared to move him, nor change the bed linen because of the agony of movement. His damaged thigh was inflamed and suppurating and, not surprisingly, he had a large bedsore. He could not sleep and he would not eat. Paré feared that the case was hopeless but nevertheless cheerfully told the patient that "by the grace of God and the help of his physicians and surgeons" he would have him on his feet again.

Having thus loyally protected his professional colleagues, he then read them the riot act. Why had they not removed the fragments of shattered bone? Why had they failed to drain and dress the wound? Why had they left him in the poisons of his filthy bed linen? They protested that the patient would not co-operate.

As Paracelsus said (about this same time): "The character of the physician may act more powerfully upon the patient than all the drugs employed." And the converse, as in this case, is true—if the doubts of the patient can dominate the physician.

Paré won the confidence of the patient. He probed, incised and dressed the wound which had been too painful to touch. He had a bed built alongside the filthy one; had it covered in spotless and fragrant linen—made it tempting for a patient, fetid in his own filth—and, after bathing him, had him lifted gently into it. He contrived a pillow to relieve the pressure on the sore.

Then he devised a shrewd contraption. He arranged a caldron into which was sprayed water from a height, freshening the air of the sickroom but also producing the effect of continuous gentle rain, a sound to soothe the patient into sleep.

He banished from the sickroom the bunkum—ground rabbit's fur and mummy powder used as dressings—and applied his "digestives." These were the mild dressings which, in his battlefield experience, he had substituted for the horrors of boiling oil and branding irons. Instead he used yolk of egg, oil of roses and oil of turpentine.

All this was what an enlightened barber-surgeon might reasonably have been expected to do—albeit Paré was the exception in his time. Where his insight becomes remarkable is in his further treatment.

They called him to dinner.

"As I came into the kitchen, I saw taken out of a great pot, half a sheep, a quarter of veal, three great pieces of beef, two fowls, and a large piece of bacon with an abundance of good herbs and I said to myself that the broth of that pot would be full of juices and very nourishing."

So he put the patient on beef extract, with raw eggs, plums stewed in wine and sugar, "and good bread, neither too fresh nor too stale, which must be got from a farmhouse." He administered mild opiates and medicines made palatable by flavorings.

The patient responded almost immediately. Soon he was enjoying the sleep which his tortured body had not had for months. Instead of praying to die, he was willing himself to live. Presently, he was approaching convalescence and Paré addressed himself to this with the same thoroughness.

"When I saw him getting well, I told him that he must have viols and violins, and a buffoon to make him laugh. Which he did."

In a month, they had him in a chair in the garden, with a hogshead of beer beside him—not for his own consumption but for the entertainment of the country people who came from far and wide to amuse him with singing and dancing. Laughter is a fine physician and six weeks after Paré took over the hopeless (i.e., without hope) case, the young marquis was walking on crutches. He then began a pilgrimage in a palanquin—not to the shrines, as was the custom, but through the villages to celebrate his recovery with the peasants whose simple frolics had been part of the cure. And the marquis drank their country beer with them "as though it had been Hippocras" (wine flavored with oriental spices).

"Dieu le guérit," said Paré—God cured him, but because a wise doctor gave him the chance, when stupid doctors, interfering—or, worse still, not interfering—misunderstood the nature of Man as they misunderstood the nature of disease.

To appreciate the real significance of this and other successes of Paré, it is necessary to remember the times in which he lived. Surgery was barbarous. On the battlefield, where Paré learned his trade, gunshot wounds were treated by pouring a mixture of boiling oil and treacle into the wounds, or by using white-hot irons to sear them. Paré escaped from this practice by accident. One night, after a battle in 1536 (during Francis I's invasion of Italy), the oil supply ran out and, as a temporary dressing, he used his "digestive" of yolk of egg, oil of roses and turpentine. Next day he went to count the dead, as a result of this failure of supplies, and found that, while those whom he had been able to scald were running temperatures, having convulsions and bleeding afresh, those who had received his improvised treatment were resting peacefully. Thenceforth he banished from his own practice all boiling oil and cautery, substituting medicamented dressings, clean bandages and clear spring water. He developed ligatures—tying cut arteries to prevent bleeding—and introduced medical orderlies to ensure that while God was curing the patient there was always someone to lend a hand.

Paré, a man of deep compassion, became the idol of the soldiers. By modern standards his methods were ruthless enough because he had no anesthetics with which to deaden the pain of amputations, and although he got as near asepsis as possible in the unhygienic conditions of his time the suffering and mortality from infected wounds were very high. Yet the soldiery exposed to such sufferings recognized in him the "good doctor." He spoke the common language, not that of the academics, and he didn't try to bewilder them with quackery or mystify them with superstition. His was not faith healing. It was faith-in-healing.

He also did his best to help the crippled. His artificial limbs were functionally useful. One of them, a mechanical hand, was based on the knight's gauntlet. In an age when it was enough merely to heal wounds without worrying about appearances, Paré went to great lengths to reduce disfigurement. He used delicate surgical instruments and adhesives to hold closed the lips of a wound for stitching, so that the scarring was reduced.

Paré, as a surgeon, refused to carry arms or to fight, although he never shirked a battle. During the persecutions of the Huguenots, although he was the surgeon of a Catholic king, he rejected royal instructions to go to Mass. He attended Admiral Coligny, the Huguenot leader, when he was mortally wounded and was himself saved from death by the king in the massacre of St. Bartholomew. For such reasons he has been claimed as a pacifist and a Protestant. The truth would appear to be that he was simply a doctor who set his service to mankind above any creed.

6. CIRCULATION OF THE BLOOD

"What," asked Robert Boyle, the great scientist, of his contemporary William Harvey, "were the things that induced you to think of a *Circulation of the Blood?*"

Harvey answered that he took notice that the valves in the veins of so many parts of the body were so placed that they allowed free passage of the blood towards the heart, but prevented the blood of the veins going the opposite way. And he had come to the conclusion that Nature had not placed so many valves without a design. So he pondered over the design and decided that the blood must be sent through the arteries and returned through the veins.

The fact that blood circulates is now so obvious that it is difficult to realize that until the year 1616 this was not generally recognized.

The Chinese had known it 4,300 years before. Hippocrates had almost guessed it when he described the blood vessels as "all of them but branches of an original vessel." He actually used the term "the circulation of the blood." Galen went astray about this and saddled succeeding centuries with his misconceptions. Vesalius, by direct observation, almost made the discovery, but, like Leonardo da Vinci, had a Galenic blind spot. So did Fabricius, of Padua, who demonstrated the fact that the valves in the veins were intended to direct the blood towards the heart, but instead of thinking of a circular motion took this to confirm Galen's notion of a kind of blood-tide—an ebb and a flow.

So it was left to Dr. William Harvey (1578-1657) to follow through the logic which they had resisted. Fabricius had been his teacher in Padua, where he, a Kent yeoman's son, had gone after leaving Cambridge. He had heard his master describe the valves as the "doors of the veins" and had made his own studies by dissection. On his return to London he became a lecturer at St. Bartholomew's hospital, where for fourteen years, he pursued his studies of the blood system. He dissected over eighty different types of animals. He noted that in addition to the valves of the veins which ensured the flow back toward the heart, the valves, or one-way doors, at the beginnings of the great arteries did the exact opposite— forced the blood away from it. He noticed two other things: that there was a bulkhead in the heart which prevented the passage of blood from one side to the other, and that the left side of the heart expelled from itself at least two ounces of blood each time it beat. This blood must go somewhere to make room for more.

By April 16, 1616, Harvey was ready to make the pronouncement which he realized was so contrary to traditional acceptance that he "trembled lest he have mankind at large for his enemies, so much doth wont and custom become a second nature."

He pinned his trust in his love of truth and he declared it to be true that the blood, forced by the action of the left side of the heart into the arteries, was distributed to the body at large and to the lungs, impelled by the right side of the heart into the pulmonary artery and then through the veins back to the left ventricle. In this way the blood flowed from the heart through the body via the arteries and back to the heart through the veins. He showed too that there was a smaller cycle with the blood moving from the right chamber of the heart to the lungs and from the lungs back to the left chamber and out into the body again.

This was one of the great turning points in medical history. Once the mechanics of the blood movement were known, men began to think of the traffic system of the body by which nutriment, oxygen, body chemicals, and indeed conditions of disease could be transported from one part of it to another. They could begin to imagine how disease could be tackled from within the body as well as from outside.

Apart from dethroning the heart from its Aristotelian sovereignty over the thoughts and the emotions and reducing it to a muscular pump whose function was to force the blood through a plumbing system, Harvey dared to investigate the mechanism of sex and processes of life creation. His book on "animal generation" was not as conclusive in its effects as that on blood circulation, but he touched on the core of the matter when he maintained that the organism did not exist encased and preformed in the ovum but evolved by gradual building up and aggregation of its parts. Others, like Fallopius, Vesalius's successor at Padua and teacher of Harvey's teacher Fabricius, had defined the system of the ovaries. That, however, had not demolished the idea of the invisible manikins who somehow grew into the unborn child, whom Leonardo had so accurately portrayed in the womb.

Harvey's ideas of the mechanism were imperfect. That was not his fault, because only with the discovery and improvement of the microscope could the processes of fertilization, and cell division and the transfer of the hereditary factors in the chromosomes and genes, be investigated. He could not determine, nor testify to, what he could not see, and he was forced to misleading analogies —saying, for example, that the fertilization of the ovum was "as iron touched by a magnet is endowed with its own powers." Not until 1875 was it proved (by Oscar Herwig, 1849-1922) that the male sperm entered the ovum and that the male and female cells combined, to divide, re-form and multiply.

7. THE REVEREND GILES EXAMINES THE BODY

In the year 1647, the Reverend Giles Firmin delivered the first lectures on anatomy in Massachusetts. How much *could* he have known (Oliver Wendell Holmes is skeptical about how much he actually *did* know) about the human body? Let us take the bits and pieces and compose a body.

He could have known all about the bones of the skeleton. He would know as much (apart from fancy names) as his Stone Age ancestors had known as they inquisitively examined the clean-picked remains of one of their fellows. As a cleric, he might have had some difficulty in explaining the continued presence of the rib which was removed to create Eve, or the missing "Luz" bone in the spinal column by which the body was to be lifted up at the Resurrection. But he would be safe with the skeleton.

Since he knew his Vesalius, he would have a useful idea of the muscles. He might know how they worked but not why. He would know the location of the principal organs but would have pretty confused ideas about their functions. He had studied Fallopius and Fabricius and would know about the blood vessels. Since he had been a student in Europe he must have known about Harvey and the blood circulation, although, even then, Harvey's "heresies" were still being hotly assailed and Firmin would be cautious, if not reticent, about the new discovery. Harvey's book on generation was not published until 1651, but Fallopius had provided material for discussion on the generative organs—if, as is unlikely, a clerical anatomist would have wanted to tackle the subject.

At least he had a skeleton, clothed in muscle and fitted with organs, and with a reproductive system which was not a complete mystery.

But (pause there) he would know nothing of the central nervous system, although he might surmise that the brain was the "control room" and not just a radiator for cooling the heart as Aristotle had supposed. Nor would he know about the digestive system. Nor the glandular system, distilling the chemicals of the body. Nor about the processes which thermostatically control the heating of the body, convert the fuel foods into energy or the protein foods into repair and maintenance materials. He might properly be preoccupied about the soul, but he would know little (unless Paracelsus had illumined him) about the interplay of mind and will and emotion on the organic functioning of the body.

In short, the Reverend Giles Firmin would know in 1647 no more than the rest of his contemporaries—that the body was a framework, a parcel wrapped in skin but in mystery as well.

And forty years later, in Salem, Cotton Mather, of Harvard, would still say: "Sickness is in fact the whip of God for the sins of man," and instigate the deaths of twenty people and torture fifty-five others into confession of the crime of witchcraft.

Part Five

THE GREAT ADVANCES (II)

> What a piece of work is a man! how
> noble in reason! how infinite in faculty!
> in form and moving how express and
> admirable! in action how like an angel!
> in apprehension how like a god! the
> beauty of the world! the paragon of
> animals!
>
> —SHAKESPEARE, *Hamlet*, Act II,
> Scene ii

1. MIND OR BRAIN?

Lord Adrian won the Nobel Prize for his experimental
work on the brain and nervous system. I once asked him:
"What is the difference between the mechanical, or electronic, brain, and the brain which conceived the mechanical, or electronic, brain?" He patiently explained the
similarities and the differences, physically, between them,
and stressed the limitations of the faculties of a computer,
compounded of valves, or transistors, and electric circuits. But, he said, the answer to my question could be
found only by a philosopher and not by an experimental
scientist.

What my question did was to confuse "mind" and
"brain." Or did it? Is our mind inside our head, like the
organ which is the brain, or is it just a figure of speech,
like the poet's idea of the heart as the seat of the emotions? After all, Aristotle gave the same sort of pre-
eminence to the heart that we give to the brain and regarded it as the center of intelligence as well as the *psyche*
or soul. Perhaps because in the last fifty years we have
discovered so much about the brain, with its 10,000,000,-
000 cells, and the marvels of the central nervous system,
we may be making a similar mistake. As Lord Adrian
put it: "Is the mind free to decide for itself, or is it tied
up with the machinery of the brain so that it can have no
independent existence or freedom?"

The brain controls all the actions of the body which

need intelligence and memory. It is the control board which signals to the muscles when, and with how much force, to contract when a skilled movement has to be made. It is the receiver of the signals which make us aware of the world around us. Like a television camera the eyes pick up the signals which form the pictures of the external world once - they are recorded by the brain cells. The ears are the microphones through which sounds are communicated to become the electrical impulses which, again, are assembled, articulated and stored, as memory, by the brain cells. The nose picks up the fine molecules of aromatic chemicals and somehow (we do not know how) changes them into signals which the olfactory nerves convey to, and register on, the cells of the brain. The taste buds of the tongue similarly react to chemical effects which again become electrical impulses conveyed to the brain. The senses of touch and pain are other electrical systems which communicate the external world to the internal brain.

All these have been measured and, with the exception of the senses of smell and taste, have been reproduced, in greater or lesser degree, by instruments in everyday use. The movie camera and the television set constitute a passable imitation of the optical nervous system. The microphone, the hi-fi phonograph disks and VHF radio are faithful reproductions of the faculty of hearing. Engineers have made instruments which, in accuracy of response, excel the human senses of touch. The electronic computer (because addition, subtraction, multiplication and division are functions of memory) has storage systems, in the form of valves or transistors, magnetic drums, or ferro-cubes which correspond to the memory cells of the brain.

While the upper brain is free from all the menial tasks of the body, the lower brain regulates the body's functions. It is the major-domo, or steward, who takes care of all the domestic chores and leaves the higher brain centers to perform more advanced activities.

The interplay of the internal, or domestic, reactions of the body has its counterpart in the automation processes of our industrial practices. The "feedback," the "servo-motors" and the automatic "programing" are the electronic engineers' version of the responses of the nervous system.

We possess, therefore, undisputable evidence of the physical faculties which are vested in the brain. A baby has to learn to walk, use his hands and learn to speak. If the appropriate parts of the brain are defective, it will never learn these things. But is learning thinking? We are back at the question whether mind and brain are one and the same thing.

The brain is often described as the organ of the mind. If the physical functions of the brain are interrupted by a knock on the head or by an anesthetic, we lose consciousness and our mind does not return until the brain has recovered. There is no doubt at all that the brain must be working properly if the mind is to take charge. But when we begin to talk of the mind and how it comes into the picture thought itself boggles.

Let us take an example. What goes on inside our skull when somebody asks a question and we give the right answer? Our ears relay the question to the brain in a code made up of electrical impulses along the nerves. The code, we know, is fairly simple and over 50,000 nerve fibers are needed to convey all the inflections of the voice. This to the sound engineer is absurd. Any of his telecommunication systems is infinitely more efficient than that. But then, a single nerve fiber is a poor signaling device compared with a telephone wire.

When we answer the question, signals go in the same way from our brain to our lips and our vocal cords which shape the right words and utter them as sound. Now if the question or answer had no meaning and we were simply repeating a sound—in at the ear and out of the mouth—the function of the brain would be clear: it would be merely a relay station between our ear and our vocal muscles. But that is not what happens. When we answer a question, the signals from the ear are sorted out and interpreted as words with a particular meaning; they are referred to some other department and evaluated and quite a different response is given by the speech muscles.

We know where the first set of signals comes into the brain and we know where the second set leaves the brain, but we still do not know what happens in between. Yet a great deal is happening there. Electrical and chemical changes are taking place all the time in the brain and have to be constantly nourished with sugar and oxygen to provide the energy for the 10,000,000,000 "radio

tubes" which are the brain cells. We do not know, there
fore, what are the mechanics of *reason*.

Nor do we know, in the scientific sense of being abl
to measure it, what constitutes *imagination*. Nor the elec
tric circuits of *moral or ethical judgment*.

2. BLUEPRINT OF LOVE

Obviously, in common experience, you cannot separat
mind and emotions. Something is known about the me
chanics of the *emotions*—how, for instance, nervou
reactions to fright or fear release chemicals from th
glands, excite the beating of the heart or give us goose
pimples. The scientist could give you a very convincin
blueprint, flow sheet or electrochemical circuit of love
But it would be just that—a prototype of the standar
mechanism, with no individual reference to the prefer
ences of the 2,500,000,000 people in the world, nor t
the vital statistics of Marilyn Monroe, nor to the seduc
tive aromas of a siren's scent, nor the romantic impulse
of moonlight in June.

For the emotions, and the complicated processes of be
havior, belong not to the electrochemists who study th
mechanism of the nervous system but to the psychologist
and psychiatrists, who have to consider not only the in
dividual but also his relations to other individuals.

In the electrochemical system of the nerves and brain
great deal has been discovered because we have becom
"communications-minded" in recent years—just as, in th
"machine-minded" nineteenth century, there were ad
vances in those aspects of physiology which dealt wit
the interchanges of work and energy. The body, to th
psychologist of the nineteenth century, was a machine
with a furnace which needed fuel in the form of food
the muscles and limbs were power tools, the heart was
pump, and so on.

A glimpse of the geography of the nervous system wa
given by Sir Charles Bell, the Scottish anatomist, at th
end of the eighteenth century. He studied the spinal cor
and found that when a nerve root was touched in the spin
muscles in the back were convulsed.

Luigi Galvani (1737-98), of Bologna, whose name
perpetuated in the "galvanometer," had started a chai
of discovery of body electricity with his famous frog's leg

xperiment. He and Lucia, his wife, chose a stormy eve-
ing to hang a dead frog by its leg with a copper wire
rom an iron balustrade. Sure enough, as the storm ap-
roached the dead frog started to twitch and convulse.
'urther experiments convinced them that they had wit-
essed a form of electricity derived from the body proc-
sses and not from the atmosphere. Indeed they had not;
hat had happened was that the suspended frog swaying
1 the wind had come in contact with the iron bars be-
ween which and the copper wire a current had been gen-
rated. It had shown the electrical aspect of nervous
timulation.

When Volta showed that similar electricity could be
enerated by copper and zinc sheets piled on top of each
ther, the result was the invention of the electric battery,
ut Galvani's animal electricity had no immediate effect
xcept to give a fresh boost to Dr. Mesmer's "animal
lagnetism," and the cult of mesmerism.

There is still argument about the way in which animal
ectricity is generated. That it is generated is beyond
oubt—as anyone who has handled an electric eel knows
) his cost. The biochemist finds a complicated substance,
cetylcholine, associated with those electrical changes,
nd it is evident that there is a chemical-electrical phe-
omenon that produces a nerve current which travels at
bout 300 feet a second.

During the nineteenth century, with instruments which
ere crude compared with those now available, experi-
lenters were nevertheless able to show, not only that all
ving tissue is sensitive to electric currents, but that all
ving tissue generates small voltages which change con-
derably when tissue is damaged or becomes active.

With something of a shudder, one recalls that the first
ectrical experiments on the brain were carried out on
le battlefield, at the battle of Sedan in 1870. Two Prus-
an medical officers, Fritsch and Hitzig, decided to test
le effect of a galvanic current on the exposed brains of
)me of the casualties, and found that, when parts of the
ft side of the brain were touched with an electrode,
lovements took place in the muscles on the right side of
le body and vice versa.

The discovery that the brain itself generated minute
ectric currents was made by an English doctor, R. Caton,
1 1875. In 1913, Prawdwicz-Neminski produced graphic

records of pulses from a dog's brain. But, because th
charges are very small and there was, then, no amplifi
cation system, the experiments could only be made on th
exposed brain and the effects were imperfect and ab
normal.

3. THE HUNGRY DOG

In 1910, Ivan Petrovitch Pavlov (1849-1936), who ha
already been awarded the Nobel Prize in 1904, likene
the nervous system to a telephone exchange. His analog
was based on the reactions of his hungry dog. He coul
make its mouth water in expectation of food via smell, o
the ringing of a bell, quarter tones on a violin, reaction
to pain, discrimination of metronome beats under or ove
100 per minute, or sound vibrations up to 120,000 pe
second. These were "conditioned reflexes," as compare
with "unconditional reflexes," which are the instincts
"Conditioning" means an association of reactions. By al
ways ringing a bell just before giving meat to a dog, Pav
lov conditioned the animal so that the sound alone wa
enough to produce a flow of saliva.

In further experiments it was found possible to con
dition dogs to discriminate between two musical notes b
giving meat after one and not after the other. If the dif
ference between the notes was too small and the nervou
system did not know whether to release saliva or not
the dogs became very excited and developed what woul
be called "neurosis" in man. The same thing can happe
today to the elaborate electronic computers. If they ge
wrong or confused signals, they will "throw a tantrum
and start behaving "neurotically."

The analogy of the brain and nervous system to a tele
phone exchange becomes all the closer as the engineer
develop more efficient automatic exchanges. The brain i
the central exchange dealing with external and interna
calls. It relays information (which, to the communica
tions engineers, are just an aggregation, and grouping, o
signals) received through the senses—eye, ear, touch
taste and smell. If the information requires judgment o
decision it will be referred to the conscious mind—(Ther
we are again! What is "brain" and where is "mind"?)—
for action.

But, sometimes, habit replaces judgment. Pavlov's do

did not reason: "The last time I heard F-sharp I got a savory steak. I shall make my mouth water in readiness." What happened was that the musical note was automatically referred to the nerves of the salivary glands, like a dialed telephone call selecting the right circuit. This can happen at a series of levels—at a series of sub-stations. For example, I am writing this. My mind is fully occupied with words and my brain is (more or less) automatically selecting the letters on the typewriter keyboard. The dog, under my desk, rubs against my leg. Without any conscious act, I draw my leg away. It resents this as unfriendly and rubs again and, without any interruption of my train of thought, I will reach down and find what is there. I am still concentrating when the dog repeats the rubbing and it becomes a conscious distraction. This time I either pat it or push it away to remove the distraction.

Each of these responses has acted through different sub-exchanges. The first time the dog rubbed, the nerve impulses got through to the "exchange" in the spine which controls the muscles which bend the knee. The leg shifted away. The same thing happened again, but this time the signal reached a more remote "exchange" which controls the arm movement. But each time there was a "spill-over"—mild impulses to the brain itself—which became cumulative and finally produced an awareness, and provoked the conscious act.

This is illustrated by reaction to pain. The finger touches something hot. The local "exchange" immediately activates the muscles and withdraws the finger. But the "fire alarm" of pain gets through to the brain and produces an awareness of hurt.

Even this is not straightforward. Take the case of the "phantom limb." People who have had limbs removed—a leg amputated above the knee, for instance—can have a sensation "in" the big toe that is not there. It is quite precise; they are aware that it is the big toe although they are also aware that the big toe does not exist. Where, then, is the seat of pain? Obviously it is not in the toe, once it has been removed. Is it in the stump? Is it in the spine? Is it in the brain? A person with a "phantom limb" can "stun" the pain by hammering the nerve endings in the stump. A local anesthetic in the appropriate part of the spine would also remove the pain. So would a narcotic acting on the brain. But so, also, if the toe actually existed would a local anesthetic in the toe. So there are whole series of exchanges controlling sections and interrelated. But that still does not explain where we *feel* pain.

The converse of all this is shock. If someone is badly injured or badly burned the shock can kill, even before the loss of blood, the organic damage, or the poisons from the burns can have their effect. An analogy is what would happen in an air raid. A whole lot of bomb "incidents" have taken place. Everyone rushes to the telephone to call Civil Defense headquarters, whose job would be to alert all the services. But because everyone is telephoning at once the central exchange is jammed with calls, cannot collect the information and cannot give instructions. In a case of shock the most elementary nerve services —like those that automatically control the temperature of the body—break down. The onslaught of external signals "jams" the internal "telephone exchange."

4. THE GEOGRAPHY OF THE BRAIN

All this does not really explain the brain, let alone the mind. It is only in recent years that the medical scientists have come to grips with this complicated organ. Before that the brain, in the map of the body, was as vague as Antarctica still is on the map of the world. Indeed the various parts were identified by the names of their explorers—the Fissure of Sylvius, the Island of Reil, the Bridge of Varolio, the Area of Broca, the Gate of Monro, the Circle of Willis. They identify as much of the cortex as can be recognized by surgical dissection, but they do not explain the behavior of the living brain.

The study of that belongs to the last thirty years. Research took the behaviorism of Pavlov and tried to blueprint it as a mechanism of cerebral events. In 1928 Hans Berger developed a method for investigation of electrical brain activity. He adapted to the brain techniques which had already served the heart specialists—through the electrocardiogram, which records the electric impulses generated by the heart as wavy ink lines on a chart.

He wanted to study the brain within the unopened casket of the skull. At first he inserted silver wires under the patient's scalp. Later he used silver foil bound to the head with a rubber band. One electrode fashioned in this way he applied to the forehead and the other to the back of the head. These he connected to a galvanometer, which in turn made ink zigzags on a piece of paper. With this relatively crude apparatus he could measure a change of one ten-thousandth of a volt. This was the beginning of the electroencephalograph, or E.E.G., now a tool of the brain surgeon and the psychiatrist as well as the brain research worker.

5. BRAIN WAVES

His basic discovery was the "Berger rhythm." He had observed that the larger and more regular variations tended to stop when the subject opened his eyes or solved some problem in mental arithmetic. With improvements in apparatus this provided a base line for the study of erratic behavior in the brain. Disease caused variations in the rhythmic oscillation and methods were developed, together with exact measurements of the geography of the brain, which enabled E.E.G. to locate tumors, lesions, and other injuries. The standard E.E.G. machine has eight channels, each of which picks up electric signals, amplifying them and operating pens to draw lines on a chart. From the complexity of zigzags, the experts can get much precise information. There is now no question that the electricity thus detected arises in the brain cells themselves.

A research refinement of the ink graph is a system of miniature television tubes which flash as the signals come through from the various parts of the brain. Thus there is projected a flickering map of the brain.

Here is the interplay of the sciences. The electronic engineers learn the nature of reflexes and feedback from the physiologists, and they in turn borrow the experience and the instruments of the engineers. The flow charts of automation imitate the nerve and muscle systems of the body and the body itself becomes intelligible from what we learn in electronic and factory engineering. The electronic computer capable of doing in split seconds complicated calculations which would take an ace mathematician months of pencil-and-paper work, is one of the great achievements of modern ingenuity.

All right! It has the ability to reproduce, and to improve

upon, nature, in one faculty of the brain, that of counting. The computer, put in charge of routine processes, can also "direct" them—it will keep them strictly in line with the instructions which have been supplied to it; but it can take no initiative and form no judgments. It has no "will," no imagination, and no powers of reasoning; those are provided by the human minds which present them to the machine as "programed information." Its not to reason why but to accept orders and impose absolute discipline on its robot slaves.

6. BUILDING A BRAIN

This sort of instrument is sometimes called an "electronic brain." But let us consider just what would be involved in the actual reproduction of a brain (leave "mind" out of it, for the moment) in terms of the most minute transistor valves. They would be no bigger than the nail of the little finger—or smaller. We would need 10,000,000,000 of them. Contracting for quantity, we might get them at ten cents each. That is $1,000,000,000 for a start.

A nerve fiber is not just a connecting wire. It is a very complicated circuit. It must carry an impulse in both directions and that impulse must travel any distance without decreasing its volume or voltage and it must conduct that impulse wherever the voltage is applied. To reproduce that circuit and wire it into the circuit of the brain, connecting up all the cells, would cost thirty million, million, million dollars, at two cents a connection. To provide power for the transistors, even with their minimal consumption, would mean a million kilowatts and the whole contraption would need a building the size of a bomber-base hangar. Contrast that with the human brain: it is about eight inches in length and about four inches in height and weighs about three pounds. It generates its own power—about 25 watts, enough to light a bedside reading lamp.

And when we had spent all those millions of millions of millions of dollars we would still not have achieved what nature has produced over millions of years and what has been functioning as the brain of Thinking Man for tens of thousands of years. We would still not have answered that question which I put to Lord Adrian—"What is the difference between the electronic brain and the brain which conceived that electronic brain?"

We might have taught it how to learn things and, by rote, to repeat what it had learned—given it memory and reason-by-association, logic, if you like, but not imagination or moral judgment. In other words we could not give it a "mind."

7. EXPLORING THE BRAIN

That is why we have *brain science* and *mental science*. There are neurophysiologists, neurophysicists and neurosurgeons and neurology—concerned with the various aspects of the brain and nervous system. But we also have psychologists and psychiatrists who are concerned with the mind and the emotions. The border line between their functions is sometimes not clear.

Obviously, physical factors in the brain can cause emotional and mental disturbances—an injury, or an obstruction or a tumor—and surgical intervention to remedy these may alter the mental state of the patient. Again, there is no doubt that *convulsive therapy* produces remarkable results (although it is often abused) on sick minds. Yet this effect is a physical one—whether it be the original injection of camphor given by Weidkhard in 1798, or the insulin shock of later years or, since 1937, the passage of electrical currents through the brain. These interventions produce man-made shocks to the brain which somehow, in many cases, fuse the split mind together.

There is *frontal leucotomy,* the values of which were nearly lost because it was too frequently employed in unsuitable cases and with imperfect experience. As a result of the systematic study of animal experiments and observation of the effect of brain damage on human behavior, it has been possible to map the brain into a number of areas which control our movements, sensations, and impressions. It has been found that there exists a "silent zone" in the forepart of the brain, which is not concerned with functions but is thought to be the region of the higher mental processes. These frontal regions are supposed to be the meeting place between the emotional impulses, arising in the lower, older part of the brain, acting on, and reacting to, the gland system, and the intellectual activities of the higher brain cells. There are masses of white fibers linking the two parts. Frontal leucotomy consists of dividing or cutting these fibers so that there is an interruption or modification of those emotional impulses.

The best results are remarkable. Patients so mentally disordered as to be certifiably insane have, by this operation, been delivered from the violent emotion, anxiety or despair which had made them a danger to themselves or others. A convincing proportion of patients treated have been able to return home and resume their normal occupations a few weeks after the operation. But this intervention does change the personality. The patient will be able to do what he has been accustomed to do, but is likely to have lost initiative and enterprise. He is likely to be placid and imperturbable, but insensitive also to the feelings of others, to the point of being embarrassingly frank, or rude, or antisocial. There is a character change wrought by the surgeon's knife.

8. REPAIRING THE BRAIN

Brain surgeons now have opportunities to carry out operations which would have been inconceivable as well as impossible only a few years ago. They can penetrate the brain with the confidence with which they might cut a muscle. This is due not only to the better charting of the brain but to advances in surgical methods and practice.

Modern aseptic routines—the absolute guarantee, under operating conditions, that no germ will ever enter the portals of the brain—was a main prerequisite. The other was the need to prevent bleeding which would injure tissue or cause clots. This has been achieved by the electric "knife," an electrode which simultaneously parts and seals the blood vessels—a humane form of cautery—and by the use of clot-preventing chemicals, the anticoagulants like *heparin* and *dicoumarin*.

The first of these was derived originally from dog liver —and Professor Charles Best, of Toronto, joint discoverer, with Frederick Banting, of insulin, played a big part in its discovery. The second is a substance which occurs in improperly cured sweet-clover silage and which has been a cause of fatal bleeding in cattle. Link, of the U.S.A., after seven years' research isolated and synthesized the agent which caused the bleeding. Its vice became a virtue. It can reduce the risk of clots which can block blood vessels.

Another great advance was the deployment of a whole range of anesthetics.

Then there was the strange story of *hypothermia*. This is artificial hibernation, or controlled freezing of the body. It was a familiar truth that hibernating animals functioned at a low body temperature, that their blood supply flowed more slowly and they consumed less oxygen. Their brains received just the minimum amount of oxygenated blood. The brain is "heavy on oxygen." The sensitive cells of highest development will die if deprived of oxygen for a very short time. The tougher cells, those which we share with the non-intellectual animals, survive longer. There have been cases where patients have "died" on the operating table, in the sense that their hearts have stopped beating. By modern methods they have been "brought back to life," but, when the delay has been more than that critical period of oxygen deficiency, the thought-process cells have withered and they have been left like zombies, walking corpses.

The problem therefore was to keep the blood flowing in just sufficient quantities, and for long enough, to allow the surgeon time to penetrate deeply into the brain. That was made possible by *hypothermia,* cooling the body to slow down the flow. This has been done by drugs, or by actually placing the patients in ice, or by pumping the blood from the heart through a mechanical cooler and back into the body again. By keeping the body at this low level of activity, the surgeons have been able to reach, and repair, parts of the brain which had been regarded as unapproachable.

9. ATOMS ON THE BRAIN

With the coming of atomic energy, new assistants have been recruited by the brain specialists—the radioactive isotopes. These can help to detect tumors deep within the brain. Neurosurgeons have for many years used certain dyestuffs to stain and identify brain tissue. When isotopes became available from atomic reactors, medical scientists tagged radioactive iodine on to one of those dyes. Since malignant cells are more greedy than normal cells they will absorb more of the dyes and be more radioactive.

Scintillator-counters can pick up the emissions from the dye and, if they are highly sensitive, may locate the tumor in its hiding place. Or radioactive potassium may be used. Another ingenious device is to embody in the affinity-dye a radioactive chemical which emits positrons —atomic particles which fly off at 180 degrees to each other. With detectors on opposite sides of the head, it is possible to plot the direction of the rays and the junction of the angle of 180 degrees will give the point of origin and the location of the tumor.

Atomic radiations can be used in treatment, either by isotopes or by beamed particles, which, with a precision greater than X rays, will pin-point the spot requiring treatment. Such needle rays have been used to reach and treat the pituitary gland, buried deep at the base of the brain. The brain has already been compared to the "Unknown Continent" of Antarctica. The activity and discoveries there during the International Geophysical Year have been no greater than the search and disclosures which have come from the exploration of the brain. Literally and metaphorically, it has been opened up.

But even that does not solve the enigma of what is *brain* and what is *mind*.

10. THE MIND DOCTORS

We had better, then, have a look at the mind doctors. In the distant past it was obvious that the emphasis of the priest-physician and the witch doctor was on the mind rather than on the body. Their treatment was primarily directed in the hope that if the patient's mind could be restored to health the body would follow suit. And so illness was explained in terms of demon possession, and the first thing to do before you tried to treat the body was to get rid of the intruder. As modern medicine develops, that ancient view becomes less ludicrous than our fathers would have supposed. More and more emphasis is being laid today upon the combined influences of mind and body.

The psychopathic patient is not unlike one who is in the power of a devil. Something is not only besetting his mind but is interfering with the proper working of his body. The doctor is all too familiar with the patient who comes to him with actual physical troubles, such as head-

ches or indigestion, and then returns with symptoms of
a quite different kind. He suggests that his physical condition is "getting him down" and that he is depressed and
losing his powers of concentration, that he is not able to
carry on his work. In the next phase he blames every-
body around him for his troubles. His family, his doctors
and his friends are all conspiring to prevent him from
getting well. And progressively his condition deteriorates
as though there was some sort of possessing force within
him which was gradually taking control of his mind and
of his body.

During the Middle Ages, the Church took the view that
illness was a punishment for sin and that its proper treatment lay in penance and prayer rather than in physical
treatment, and special rituals and services were devised
for the casting out of devils. This could act as a psychological shock treatment, often with beneficial results not
only to the mind but to the body. Thus, a great deal of
the treatment in olden days and in the Middle Ages was
in fact psychotherapy.

As medicine became scientific, however, and began to
recognize the functions of the body as akin to those of a
machine, less and less importance was attributed to the
mind as a cause of disease. One of the people who contributed to this tendency was the French scientist Descartes, who distinguished between the material body of man
and his immaterial mind.

The function of the doctor, as he became more and
more specialized, was to direct his attention to the patient's
body and leave his mind to others—to the theologians,
the spiritual advisers, or to the philosophers. This would
not have been so bad if the two groups—the body doctors
and the spiritual doctors—had compared notes, but instead there was a complete divorce between their attitudes
and their ideas. And when there is a division of interests
in this way there is, in the no man's land between, plenty
of room for quacks who can exploit both sides.

1. MESMERISM

It is very difficult to decide whether Franz Anton Mesmer
(1733-1815) was in fact the rogue and charlatan which
the physicians of his time thought him to be.

Mesmer, like Paracelsus, was convinced that man was

influenced and deflected by forces which reached him from other parts of the universe. He was born in Switzerland and studied medicine, taking his medical degree in Vienna in the year 1766. He chose for his thesis the theme of the influence of the planets on the human body. Through a Jesuit professor of astronomy, Mesmer became interested in experiments with magnets. He tried magnets in a case of heart disease with apparent benefit to his patient. Later he formed the theory that since everything in the universe was common, and there was a universal "mobile fluid," his own body must be possessed of magnetism, and that the effects he had produced or appeared to have produced with magnets could be achieved by the hand alone.

By magnetic influence or what we now call mesmerism through the hands, Mesmer appeared to have remarkable successes. These brought him into violent conflict with the orthodox doctors of Vienna and finally he went to Paris where he became a fashionable success, one of the "lions" of high society. He had so many patients that he could not cope with them and invented various devices by which he was supposed to have transferred his power to pieces of iron.

A Parisian commission appointed to investigate Mesmer's claims conceded that he had brought about many cures but denied the existence of such a thing as "animal magnetism." This is a vague term and most doctors today would probably agree with the verdict of the commission, but might suggest that there was in Mesmer's cures an element of what has since associated "mesmerism" with hypnosis.

This was borne out by the experience of one of Mesmer's disciples who was more scientific than his master. He made three observations: That the patients who reacted well to mesmeric treatment heard only what the magnetizer said to them and took in nothing else; that they accepted his suggestions without questioning them; that they could recall nothing of what happened after their return to normal consciousness. This we would now recognize as hypnotism as practiced by showmen, but also by highly reputable doctors.

It was the interest in hypnotism which led to events of great importance to modern medicine. Jean Martin Charcot (1825-93) was a world-famous physician who set up

he famous Paris hospital of the Salpetrière. He decided
o investigate the subject of hypnotism and at length
oncluded that the hypnotic state was a condition re-
embling hysteria. He was, therefore, very doubtful if it
ad any value in the treatment of abnormal psychological
tates.

2. ENTER FREUD

n 1885 a son of poor Moravian parents, who had quali-
ed as a doctor in Vienna, arrived at Charcot's hospital.
his was Sigmund Freud (1856-1939). His visit and the
npression made on him by Charcot led Freud to abandon
onventional medicine and devote himself entirely to the
eatment of nervous disorders. This coincided with the
isit of another physician to Charcot's clinic—Breuer,
ho was convinced of the values of hypnotism in the
ure of neurotic disorders. He told Freud about a young
oman patient who was suffering from partial paralysis
nd from difficulty in speech. He had put her under hyp-
osis and had questioned her about the cause of her
ouble and she had traced it back to a time when she
as under great emotional stress involving her father, to
hom she was deeply devoted. When she came out of
ie trance and the circumstances of the incident were re-
alled, her paralysis disappeared.

Freud followed up this case by researches of his own
nd decided that there were mental processes which were
uried deep and behind consciousness. These depths were
eached in the condition of hypnotism, but he discovered
1at hypnotism was not essential in order to reveal them.
Ie invented the "psychiatric couch" where, lying relaxed,
atients could be reduced to a somnolent state in which
1ey could recount the thoughts fleeting through their
1ind. In the process the "unconscious" could be tapped.
ne idea could lead to another and the patient could be
onducted quietly back through his or her past life until
1e investigator could discover the event or circumstance
hich might have caused the functional troubles. Freud
eveloped the view that in our conscious life ideas and
npulses originate in our unconscious, where they are
ally emotions which are never clearly expressed in
ords. What was of special importance to Freud was the
ct that many of these unconscious ideas and wishes

are repressed—they cannot find expression by becoming conscious.

This restraint and suppression was attributed by Freud to an "endopsychic censor" which allowed only those things of which it approved to pass over into the realm of the conscious. The idea thus repelled by the censor, or the gatekeeper of the conscious, continued its existence but, in the unconscious, rebelled and became neurosis or hysteria. He came to the conclusion that most of the deep-seated conflicts of this kind were of a sexual nature. Society had placed so many taboos on sexual behavior that sexual experience was likely to be associated with a strong sense of guilt.

His own famous disciples, Adler and Jung, were later to dispute this stress on the thwarted sexual urge as a prime cause of neurosis and there have been great conflicts of opinion on this point, regarded by so many as the basis of the Freudian creed. Adler modified the teachings of his master and drew attention to the fact that the individual encountered great difficulties in adjusting himself to society and in his efforts to secure personal power. He believed that from such things neurosis could arise. Jung suggested that nervous breakdowns generally arose from the person's incapacity to find expression for the creative impulses lying in his unconscious. Jung was also responsible for the idea of the "collective unconscious." This means the unconsciousness of the race itself in contrast to the "personal unconscious" of the individual. A well-adjusted man according to this approach was one who had found a proper balance between the race unconscious and the personal unconscious.

No amount of controversy can ever minimize the great contribution which Freud made to psychological medicine. He was the first to stress the importance of unconscious conflicts in functional diseases and to show that if those conflicts could be brought to the surface successful treatment could follow. The fact that there was a rational approach to the treatment of mental and nervous disorders was itself a very important factor influencing the attitude to the mentally sick which developed in this century.

3. MERCY FOR THE MENTAL

Throughout the ages the treatment of the insane has been barbarous. As late as the time of Dr. Samuel Johnson and James Boswell the public were allowed to make ours of Bedlam, the Bethlehem Hospital for the insane in London, to stare at the raving men and women chained to the floor or exhibited in cages.

There were compassionate people in all ages who were horror-stricken by such treatment of human beings, but it was a young French doctor, Dr. Philippe Pinel (1745-1826), who is remembered as the Crusader. One of his friends had lost his mental balance and been locked up in a madhouse. He contrived to escape from his cage and bolted to the woods, where his body was found half-devoured by wolves. This incident made Pinel vow that he would devote himself in future to the study of insanity and to the improvement of its victims.

He was convinced that the insane were sick people in need of treatment. After the French Revolution he petitioned the Commune to allow him to appear before it and to plead the citizen rights of the mentally sick. Of course, he was regarded as a madman trying to liberate madmen, but he pleaded that since all men were possessed of equal rights his poor mentally ill patients also had their rights. Yet they were kept, he pointed out, in dungeons and were treated barbarously. Pinel got his way and was allowed to give the insane freedom from their chains, but was warned that his own life would be sacrificed for this "false mercy."

Within the space of a few days Pinel had struck the chains from more than fifty men who had been regarded as dangerous madmen. They were still insane, but with kindly treatment they ceased to be rebellious and disorderly. Many enlightened doctors shared this view of Pinel that insanity was only ill health in a different form and that it could respond to decent treatment.

In America his contemporary, Benjamin Rush (1745-1813), produced one of the first systematic works on the diseases of the mind to be written in the Western world. From his earliest days as a medical student he had crusaded for more humane treatment of the insane. As a

117

result of his campaigning, decent quarters, at least, we:
built for them in Pennsylvania Hospital. One of his e:
cellent suggestions was that madmen should be treated b
occupational therapy. He suggested the setting-up of wor:
shops and spinning wheels and proposed too that the p
tients should be encouraged to meet normal people willi:
to join them in conversation, read to them and discu
their troubles. By this emphasis on persuading patients
discuss their troubles he foreshadowed the technique
modern psychoanalysis.

Rush believed that madness was in part, or in som
cases, due to overstimulation of the blood vessels of th
brain. Although this was perhaps an excuse for his ow
obsessional ideas about blood-letting, nevertheless it w
a step forward because it postulated that conditions of th
body often caused disorders of the mind.

In Britain the lead towards more humane treatment
the insane was taken by the Quakers when in the yea
1792, at the instigation of William Tuke, a home calle
The Retreat—"a place in which the unhappy might o
tain refuge"—was opened at York.

Even today, however, there is still much to be desire
in the accommodation and treatment of the mental
sick. Under the stresses of the modern world the numb
of mental cases who require hospital treatment is increa
ing to an alarming extent. On the other hand, advance
in treatment have meant that many who only a few yea
ago would have been regarded as hopeless and would ha·
been confined, for the safety of themselves and others,
a mental hospital, can in gratifyingly increasing propo
tions be restored to normal life. This largely depend
however, on early recognition and proper diagnosis of th
trouble. E.E.G. (the "brain-wave" meter), medical hy
nosis, and psychoanalysis can all help in this.

14. ALICE-IN-WONDERLAND DRUGS

Drugs, too, can help to give access to the secret places
the mind. Narcotics and "tranquilizers" can break dov
the emotional defenses and enable the psychiatrist to di
cover the cause of the disturbance. He now has at h
disposal a large range of chemicals which affect the ner
ous system and the brain in different ways and give hi
entrance into Freud's "unconscious." Worlds as weird

nose which science fiction writers discover in space are revealed, in the mind, by some of these drugs.

For example, there is the "Alice-in-Wonderland" drug, -lygergic acid diethylamide or "L.S.D. 25." It was discovered by two Swiss chemists in 1938 as a factor in ergot, a fungus that causes a disease of grains—which, incidentally, may have been one of the causes of the epidemic of Dancing Mania in the Middle Ages.

You remember the little bottle in *Alice in Wonderland* with the label that said: "Drink me." " 'What a curious feeling!' said Alice. 'I must be shutting up like a telescope!' . . . and her face brightened up at the thought that she was now the right size for going through the little door to that lovely garden."

L.S.D. 25 gives certain cases just that kind of feeling. They return through time and diminish in size—at least that is their sensation.

A married woman who was given the drug in a British Mental Hospital said: "I wondered if I had gone small and looked to see and was not the least surprised to find my arm and hand quite little, the size of that of a child of seven or eight. I did not feel small but when I looked I had shrunk. It seemed to me as if I were shopping with mother in a large store. She had walked on without my realizing it, and when I turned to speak to her, I was a little girl alone and lost."

Similarly a woman of twenty-nine felt she had diminished to a child of five or six years old. She felt her ordinary clothes loose about her, like a child playing "pretends" in a grownup's dress. The doctor's hand seemed large as an adult's hand would seem to a child.

Another woman, to whom the drug was given in her own home, remained at the apparent age of eight for a whole fortnight. Her contemporaries seemed much larger than she and her own children became her childhood playmates.

Her home became her old school and her bedroom her childhood nursery. She was living simultaneously in two periods of time.

This drug, however, is no party game. Cases have described it as a horrifying experience, not a bit like reminiscing. A minute dose of such a drug causes the real world to seem to disintegrate. Everything becomes tinged with blue or red. Walls start moving to and fro,

like trick photography in a film. Tears stream from the pa
tients' eyes, but not from emotion. They separate ou
into two personalities—one the bystander looking at an
clearly describing the child they are gradually becom
ing. They go back, stage by stage, and, as though i
confirmation of Freud, they stop at the incident in tim
which is the secret emotional event which the doctors ar
trying to uncover. They go back to "what happened i
the woodshed."

Sometimes the results are more freakish. Subjects hav
been known to report their retreat back into the woml
they have become embryos. Others have reported previou
"incarnations." One subject described very vividly a pre
vious existence in the time of the Egyptians, althoug
away from the influence of the drug, there was comple
ignorance of Egyptology. Is this, like the illusions pr
duced by mescalin and similar drugs, just hallucination
Or is it "mental speleology"—a descent into the dar
caves of the mind and a wrenching open of the locke
doors of emotional secrets? Come to that, what are "ha
lucinations" anyway? Drugs of the new tranquilizer typ
(based on the Vedantic drug rauwolfia) have produce
another revolution. Patients can now be treated at hom
instead of being hospitalized for long periods. In th
United States, where the care of mental patients costs $
billion a year, there was in 1956 a reduction for the fir
time in 184 years in the total number of hospitalize
mental cases.

Instead of a predictable 12,000 increase there was
decrease of 8,000. This meant nearly 20,000 fewer p
tients and a saving in treatment and hospital constructio
of $200 million. More and more, shock treatments, pac
and tubs, and physical restraints are being replaced
sedatives and tranquilizers.

Occupational therapy for mental conditions has gor
further even than Benjamin Rush suggested. One of th
healing processes is to encourage mental patients to pai
and in their wild excursions into color, more extravaga
than those of the most "advanced" painters, they sp
out in patterns their hallucinations in terms unmistakat
to the psychiatrist.

15. VICTORIES IN THE MIND

The success of any treatment of mental ill health depends on the recognition by the public, as well as by doctors and patients, that sickness of the mind must be accepted as matter-of-factly as the ills of the body. Otherwise we are still in the Middle Ages, believing that the unfortunate whose mind is sick is vested with demons. This escape from demonology into a rational acceptance of the mental invalid is one of the great advances of our time.

The social attitude toward mental ill health is itself therapeutic. In Holland, it has now reached the stage where a diminishing proportion of patients is confined to hospital. They are treated in their homes and at their work, and their families and work-mates take part in the treatment—they learn how to behave towards a mental casualty. This new approach—treating the mental out-patient—is very important. While hospital treatment can be effective and a patient can be discharged as cured, he or she has got to fit back into the social environment, the stresses of which had produced the original maladjustment. If "running repairs" can be carried out in the actual environment, the restoration is all the easier and the more enduring.

This is another reminder that, as is stated in the charter of the World Health Organization, "health is a state of complete physical, mental and social well-being, and not merely the absence of disease and infirmity."

Part Six

THE GREAT ADVANCES (III)

> ARE YOU SENSITIVE? Sensitive peo-
> ple are the intelligent people of this
> world. They are intense, alert—*they
> are often the indigestion sufferers*. It
> is a well-known medical fact that if
> you are sensitive, the nervous system
> of your stomach, so closely linked with
> the brain, works faster and becomes
> tense and over-wound. The answer is . . .
>
> —*From a stomach-powder advertisement*

1. ST. MARTIN'S WINDOW

Mackinac Island, at the junction of Lake Huron and Lake
Michigan, called by the Indians "The Turtle," was, on
June 6, 1822, a scene of milling excitement. The Indian
canoes were paddling furiously across the water and an
armada of French-Canadian boats was converging on the
beaches. Ashore there was feasting and singing and dancing.

There was nothing unusual about this. Those were
merely the Indians coming in to trade fur pelts for trin-
kets and whisky and the *voyageurs,* the boatmen and
porters of the fur brigades, bringing in the furs collected
in the wilderness of the West. After months in the wilds,
living on water, corn and pemmican, the *voyageurs* were
in a mood to drown a winter's thirst in firewater and to
feast and to fight.

The American Fur Company's store was crowded to
suffocation with men boastful and exuberant. In the midst
of the shouting and hubbub there was an explosion. A
gesticulating *voyageur* had accidentally triggered off his
musket. A nineteen-year-old youngster, Alexis St. Martin,
who had been within three feet of the muzzle, fell to the
floor, his body ripped open by the shot and his shirt in
flames. The shout went up to get a priest and to get a
doctor. The odds were on the priest, for St. Martin's case
seemed hopeless.

Dr. William Beaumont (1785-1853), an army surgeon from Connecticut, was called from the fort and found the youth in an apparently hopeless condition. A portion of the lung and a part of the stomach were extruding from the wound and the stomach itself was lacerated. No one, in those days, was likely to survive such injuries. Beaumont gave St. Martin twenty minutes to live. (In fact St. Martin outlived his doctor by twenty-eight years.)

Beaumont cleansed the wound and applied a superficial dressing. When the injured man survived the twenty minutes, the doctor re-dressed the wound and extracted shot, wadding and splintered bones—a process in itself calculated to speed the end. But the *voyageurs* were mighty tough people and St. Martin's body for months afterwards was expelling splintered bone and shot, and healing itself. The one thing the healing processes (in the absence of plastic surgery) could not do was to close the gaping wound, exposing the stomach. For ten months Beaumont dressed the wound and tried to close it. Then he proposed an operation, which St. Martin refused.

A year after the accident St. Martin was on his feet, still with a naked opening into his stomach. The hole in the stomach wall itself remained unclosed, but nature had contrived a kind of valve, like a tongue of a shoe, which kept the food in during the process of digestion. The poor law authorities of Mackinac wanted to ship him home to Canada, but Beaumont, believing that he would not survive the journey—2,000 miles by canoe—took him into his own home.

This was the beginning of one of the most extraordinary episodes in medical history. Beaumont was a mere frontier doctor without any experience of medical research but he realized that here he had a freak opportunity of studying the processes of digestion, which, despite the researches of Regnier de Graaf (1641-73) on the pancreatic juices, still remained a mystery.

Through the "lid" of St. Martin's stomach, he could withdraw and examine the gastric juices; he could look directly into the cavity of the stomach, observe its motion and almost see the process of digestion; he could string pieces of meat or vegetables, lower them into the stomach and withdraw them at various stages of digestion; he could use a plug of raw beef, instead of lint, to block the opening, and when he did so he found that "in less than five hours it had been completely digested off."

St. Martin, meanwhile, was working as the odd-job man around the place, and periodically would threaten to ruin the experiments by getting drunk. It was an extraordinary relationship, in which the two men on such intimate terms did not like each other. Beaumont took the young man around to medical societies like a traveling showman. And then one day, at Plattsburg, a few miles from St. Martin's native Canada, the "exhibit" disappeared. He returned to Canada, married and had children, but he could earn only a poor living and finally chose to return to Beaumont and become again an experimental animal. He and his master became famous all over the United States, and visited Europe as a showpiece for the medical societies there. When Beaumont died St. Martin set up in business on his own and hired himself out as an exhibit, but when he died his family rejected the large sum of money which Sir William Osler offered for permission to carry out a post-mortem and secure the famous stomach for a museum. They buried him in secret and at great depth.

2. DIGEST OF DIGESTION

One of the things which Beaumont discovered from this living experiment was that gastric juice appeared only when food entered the stomach or was being chewed in the mouth. For the first time he obtained pure gastric juice; he sent a sample to Professor Dunglison of the University of Virginia, who found that it contained hydrochloric acid.

From this starting point, in Alexis St. Martin's stomach and the backwoods of America, we can begin to study and understand the digestive system. We can regard it, in its most simple form, as a tube with automatic muscles. Into this tube glands along its course pour chemicals. Some of these glands are actually in the wall of the tube. Others, like the pancreas and the liver, are so large that they are constructed outside the tube and discharge their chemicals through a duct into the digestive canal. All the movements in the digestive system, whether it is the chewing in the mouth, or peristalsis—the wormlike movement by which the tube propels its contents—

or the churning motion of the stomach, are synchronized, and interdependent with the chemical system.

The movement of the jaw and of the lips, the grinding and crushing action of the teeth, and the rolling of the food by the tongue and the cheeks are associated with the secretion of saliva, the chemicals of which contribute to the preparation of the food for reception by the stomach. Mastication and swallowing are voluntary movements— we can consciously direct them—but from there on, as we often discover to our discomfort, the digestive system is automatic and beyond our control.

The stomach is a muscular sac which is separated from the intestines by a strong band of muscle called the *pylorus*. This is the "trap door" which at intervals opens to allow a well-digested lump of food to enter the duodenum (so called because it is twelve fingerbreadths in length), which is part of the small intestine.

The movements of the stomach consist of waves of contraction—squeezing—and also a churning movement. The stomach empties itself in about four hours and the process is then taken over by the intestine, which, small and large together, is twenty-five feet long. As the food moves through the coils of tubular membrane it is mixed with intestinal, pancreatic and liver juices, which convert the food into the substances the body requires and which it absorbs into the blood stream through the intestinal walls. When the food reaches the large intestine the chemical processes are virtually over and it becomes a matter of sewage disposal—the excretion of the waste products.

Digestion is a process of chemical change. The chemicals of the external world are supplied in the form of food, which is treated by the digestive juices, and the various chemicals which the body needs are sorted out and passed into the blood stream. These digestive juices are mainly enzymes, which are catalyzers. A catalyst is like a parson at a wedding ceremony; it completes a union without being involved in the combination. Two chemicals which would not spontaneously combine will do so in the presence of a catalyst which itself remains intact when the process is completed; it has changed other substances, without itself changing.

The action of most of those body enzymes is astonishingly rapid. Within five seconds a piece of bread in the mouth will turn sweet. This is due to an enzyme in the saliva called *ptyalin,* whose job it is to digest starch. This it does by breaking down the complex starches of the bread into simple sugars.

The stomach enzyme is *pepsin.* It is concerned only with proteins and albuminous foods—meat and eggs and so on. The pepsin is produced by small glands all over the walls of the stomach, but the enzyme can only act in the presence of acid. That is why the stomach glands secrete hydrochloric acid as well.

After the food leaves the stomach numerous other enzymes take over. Some of these are from glands in the wall of the intestine. The most potent of all the juices, however, are those secreted by the pancreas and poured into the upper part of the intestine. One of the pancreatic chemicals, *trypsin,* quickly breaks up protein foods. Another, *lipase,* splits fats into more easily absorbed compounds. A third of the enzymes from the pancreas is *amylase,* which carries on the job which the saliva had begun and breaks down starches and sugars into simpler chemical forms. From the Islets of Langerhans in the pancreas comes *insulin,* that vital substance which controls the absorption of sugar into the blood and the lack of which produces diabetes.

This elaborate process of mixing, breaking down, splitting up and passing on into the blood, which is the transport system of the body, takes place along the twenty feet of small-gauge intestine.

The proteins and starches are absorbed through the walls of the intestine by the network of small veins which spread over its surface. They are the tributaries which empty into larger and larger veins and are carried by the portal vein to the liver, which is the largest solid organ inside the body. One of its functions is to provide bile as one of the chemicals for the intestine, but it is also a storehouse for the starch and sugars, in the form of *glycogen.* It is also concerned with the handling of the proteins. In addition it plays a role in the blood system. The spleen destroys the outworn blood cells and the liver handles the waste. The liver is the store for the indispensable Vitamin B_{12}, the most potent physiological chemical we know, without which the body suffers from pernicious anemia, the lack of red blood cells. Another liver product is *fibrinogen,* which causes the blood to clot and form a crust for a wound; but, by way of compensation, it also produces *heparin,* which checks clotting.

There are other absorbent vessels on the surface of the small intestine which absorb mainly fat and, sometimes, any surplus protein. They are the tributaries of the lymph system, the main stream of which is the thoracic duct which runs upward along the spine and empties its contents into one of the large veins at the root of the neck.

The stomach is nearly always free from bacteria because its acid destroys most of them, but the intestines have an increasing number of germs—the large intestine swarms with them. But not all of them are malevolent. Many of them serve a useful purpose in the processes of digestion and conversion of food, and physiologists sometimes have to remind doctors who are prodigal in their use of germ-killing antibiotics that they may be interfering with the beneficial processes of nature.

3. BON APPETIT

Thus in the digestive system we have a chemical plant more impressive in its ramifications even than those of the du Ponts, Imperial Chemical Industries or I. G. Farben. But this is only part; presently we will be discussing the fine-chemical factories within the body—the endocrines.

What causes the production and secretion of the gastric juices? As Beaumont discovered, the gastric juice from the stomach appeared only when food was being chewed in the mouth or as it was actually entering the stomach. The juices, therefore, are not flowing all the time. We can see this in the case of saliva; sometimes the mouth is dry; sometimes the mouth "waters," and when we put food in the mouth it flows. This is equally true of the juices of the stomach and intestine—they appear in the presence of food.

It was the study of the salivary secretion in dogs which led Pavlov to his discovery of the conditioned and unconditioned reflexes. Left to itself a dog's mouth does not water until food is actually presented to it. Pavlov, however, rang a bell just before giving a dog food. After a time the dog's mouth would water when the bell rang, even if there was no food in sight. This was a "conditioned reflex," which means that through experience the dog had learned to associate a new stimulus with food.

Pavlov varied his experiments. He would, for example, show a dog a circular patch of light before feeding him and the dog's mouth would water at the mere sight of a circular patch. He then showed a dog an ellipse of light and every time it appeared the dog would be given an electric shock. Thus the dog learned to distinguish between circles and ellipses and to expect food in one case and shock in another. Gradually the ellipse was changed into a circle and this produced in the dog a mixture of sensations—pleasure at the sight of a circle and fear at the sight of an ellipse. If the ellipse was almost circular, the dog would have a nervous breakdown just as a human being would have in a conflicting situation which he could not resolve.

Pavlov's work on dogs has been confirmed in man. The circumstances were rather like those which offered the opportunity to Beaumont. A man's gullet had been seriously burned and to feed him the surgeons had to make a false opening into his stomach. It was thus possible to measure the amount of gastric juice produced under different circumstances. When the man smelled something which he liked to eat, the gastric juice was poured out in large quantities. When it was something which he disliked the stomach wall would be dry. Although he could not swallow, because of his damaged gullet, the chewing of food of pleasant taste produced a flow of gastric juices.

This is the sort of thing we mean by "good appetite." Unless you are starving, and the body is bereft of the external chemical (food) it needs, you will digest more of the food you swallow if it is something you like. The smell of food, the color, the "dressing," all influence the flow of the body chemicals which are necessary to convert food to its proper use.

There was a famous British music-hall artiste, Marie Lloyd, who had a song which might have earned her a Ph.D. as a physiologist: "A little of what yer fancies does yer good."

4. RASPUTIN STOMACH

The digestive system is a Klondike and a bonanza for the patent-medicine dealers. Fortunes are made from pills, from powders and draughts. Because the consumption of food, its absorption and discharge, is a commonplace function, people take liberties in self-medication. And it is true all over the world. All primitive societies have their laxatives and purgatives.

Once in the wilds of Burma I saw a medicine man, with a tall gilt hat like a pagoda, with an ornate, red leather apron and a gong, plying his trade in a village. With cant and incantation he was dispensing a cure-all. I managed to get a sample of his magic powder, had it analyzed and found that it was no better and no worse than a drugstore pill. Its basis was a local form of rhubarb, the laxative. For many of the complaints for which he was selling it, it had no specific value but no doubt served its purpose, psychologically, because the subject had an awareness of "something happening."

Yet, as we have seen, the body is very careful in its checks and balances. Enzymes and "juices" interact. If, therefore, people persistently use extraneous drugs to do the job which the digestive juices themselves should do, the normal functions will be overruled—purges will produce chronic constipation.

Today one of the commonest complaints of our high-speed overstressed civilization is "acid stomach"—an excessive amount of hydrochloric acid. This is often associated with duodenal and peptic ulcers, the trade mark of big business and the penalty of the executive suite. Antacids may relieve the complaint but may be smothering the symptoms of something much more serious. They certainly would not touch the cause of the stresses, to which we will be returning.

While some people suffer from excess of acid, a proportion of people—about five percent—have "Rasputin stomachs." This refers to the extraordinary case of the Russian monk who acquired a malevolent power over the ill-fated tsar and tsarina of Russia. A group of courtiers conspired to get rid of him, and administered a dose of cyanide, a deadly poison. Rasputin survived the cyanide (to be shot later) because his stomach did not produce hydrochloric acid. In the normal stomach, if cyanide came into contact with the acid, a gas would be given off, absorbed immediately into the blood stream and would prevent the working of oxygen in the brain and the muscles. This would cause chemical asphyxia and death would follow, as in the case of the suicide of Himmler and Goering, within two or three minutes.

Rasputin was certainly a sinister character. He exercised a mesmeric power over the tsarina, who was all the more susceptible because her son was hemophilic—(a "bleeder"); he suffered from a failure of his blood to clot, a hereditary complaint, exaggerated in royalty by the in-breeding of "royal blood." The monk was regarded by the courtiers as one in league with the devil and one can imagine the horrific confirmation of this when they found that he survived the normally deadly and instantaneous poison. But the physiology of the digestive system provides a perfectly rational explanation—a hydrochloric deficiency.

Part Seven

THE GREAT ADVANCES (IV)

> There's language in her eye, her cheek,
> her lip,
> Nay her foot speaks; her wanton spirits
> look out
> At every joint and motive of her body.
>
> —SHAKESPEARE, *Troilus and Cressida,*
> *Act iv, Scene v*

1. FAT BOY JOE

" 'Damn that boy,' said the old gentleman, 'he's gone to sleep again.'

" 'Very extraordinary boy that,' said Mr. Pickwick, 'does he always sleep in this way?'

" 'Sleep!' said the old gentleman, 'he's always asleep. Goes errands fast asleep, and snores when he waits at table.'

" ' How very odd!' said Mr. Pickwick.

" 'Ah, odd indeed,' returned the old gentleman, 'I'm proud of that boy—wouldn't part with him on any account—damme, he's a natural curiosity!' "

And a medical one! An endocrinologist reading Dickens' *Pickwick Papers* would immediately diagnose Fat Boy Joe's abnormality as *dystrophia adiposogenitalis,* or he might call it *Fröhlich's syndrome*.

His diagnosis would be reinforced by the later interlude in the book when with stealth and sinister look the Fat Boy creeps up on old Mrs. Wardle to tell her about the love passage between Mr. Tupman and Rachel:

" 'Then what can you want to do now?' said the old lady gaining courage.

" 'I want to make your flesh creep,' replied the boy."

A streak of sadism—perhaps just "teasing" like this—is another characteristic of this *dystrophia*.

If Fat Boy Joe were alive—as a boy—today, Mr. Wardle would lose his "curiosity." The doctors would put him on glandular treatment and Joe's somnolent fatness would give way to the slim alertness of any normal teen-ager. His condition was due to underactivity of the pituitary, or hypophysis, gland. This gland governs the rhythm of sleep (with its seasonal manifestation in the hibernation of animals), and a flaw in the gland can repress the proper development of the sex characteristics in a growing child and cause fatness. The balance can be restored by administering artificially the gland extracts which are deficient.

When Dickens' *Pickwick Papers* appeared, in 1837, people were not aware of the *endocrines,* those glands that produce the remarkable chemicals which dominate our physical shapes, the functioning of our organs, and our emotional behavior. Ten years later, Claude Bernard, the French physiologist, first promoted the idea of "internal secretions" when he found that there were chemicals generated within the body which controlled the amount of sugar in the blood. But in the Dingley Dell days the nearest the doctors had got to the chemistry of temperament was the Four Humors.

Back in the Middle Ages, the learned doctors of Salerno had related the "humors" of Aristotle, Empedocles and Galen to temperament and personality. They classified people by their appearance and behavior and codified those to the "humors" which were dominant.

The Sanguine Man had an excess of hot, moist blood; therefore he was inclined to be fat and prone to laughter —a jovial fellow who loved "mirth and musick, wine and women."

The Phlegmatic Man had an excess of cold phlegm; therefore he was square-built and "given to rest and sloth."

The Choleric Man had too much hot, yellow bile in his system; therefore he was a man of violent temper, "fierce, and full of fire and given to anger for little cause."

The Melancholic Man had too much dry, black bile; therefore he had a sulky, heavy look "with spirit little daring, pensive, peevish, and ever solitary."

2. THE BODY STATE

Although we still accept them adjectivally, the doctrine of the humors as a medical concept was undermined a century ago by Virchow's "cellular pathology."

Rudolf Virchow, born in Pomerania in 1821, was himself a choleric man "given to anger on little cause" and capable of scientific extravagances when roused—as when Armand de Quatrefages called the Prussians "Huns."

De Quatrefages, the famous ethnologist, was understandably angry when, during the Franco-Prussian War, German shells fell on the Paris Natural History Museum. He was so furious that he argued that the Prussians were not Nordic, not even Teutonic, but Mongols left behind by Attila.

This in turn infuriated Virchow. As a member of the Prussian House of Delegates he introduced a bill allowing him to examine ALL the schoolchildren in Prussia—six million of them. They were lined up; their heads were measured with calipers; their bone formations were examined; one hair of each head was pulled out and classified; and their teeth were inspected. And he proved scientifically that the Prussians were not Huns but Franks—like the French, only more so. But the appellation "Hun" stuck.

Absurd? But typical of the scientific thoroughness which made Virchow one of the greatest figures in medical history. Choleric, yes. But kindly too and quick to anger about inhumanity and injustice. He fed the flames of German liberalism in 1848 by producing a medical report. The government, unwisely, had sent him to investigate an epidemic of "famine fever" raging in Upper Silesia. He went and lived among the weavers, did his researches, and then produced facts which the authorities did not want to hear. The sickness of the people of Upper Silesia was no Act of God (as famine was then regarded) but typhus fever due to the filth of their stinking living conditions.

He went further: In his report he said that those suffering men and women were citizens of the great Prussian state, yet the state had neglected to provide even the most elementary protection for their welfare. So they were sick, and since they were sick, the state itself was sick. Not only must the Prussian people clean the houses of the weavers; they must fumigate the government. They must not only drive out the rats; they must smoke out the councillors. They must build not only clean houses but a clean, democratic state.

Not surprisingly he was "purged" from his government post in Prussia, but he was given a professorship at the University at Würzburg, which was prepared to accept a scientist on his academic distinction and to overlook his politics.

In his Silesian report, the "sick" individual and the "sick" state had been a young man's angry metaphor. But now he applied that metaphor to human pathology.

His argument went something like this: What makes a state prosperous? It is the prosperity of each individual citizen. What, then, makes the living body healthy? It is the health of each of its units—its cells. Disease, he contended, was anarchy within the body. As he put it in his *Cellular Pathology* (1858): "The body is a cell-state in which every cell is a citizen. Disease is merely a conflict of the citizens of the state brought about by the action of external forces."

3. CELL-CITIZENS

In the background of Virchow's ideas was the work, two hundred years previously, of Marcello Malpighi (1628-94) and of Robert Hooke (1635-1703). With microscopes, which had by then been invented, Malpighi had examined and described the structure of the tissue of the body and Hooke, working with plants, had described "little boxes or cells, distinct from one another."

In the interval it had been recognized that the different organs were different because they were formed from different kinds of cells. Virchow, with his improved microscopes, and with a device by which the body tissue could be cut into strips so thin that they were transparent to light and when stained with blue dye revealed their cell structure under the microscope, would take an abscess of the lung, which to the naked eye was white and ugly and "diseased," and would show it under the microscope to consist of a mob of white cells, just like the leucocytes of normal blood. The cells were just wandering cells of an unhealthy body-state. He examined cancer of the skin and found that its cells were just like the neighboring, and normal, skin cells, except that they looked even more fresh and vigorous. If he had lived to see his Germany under Hitler, he might have, in his metaphor, compared them to the Nazi storm troopers, physically sound but antisocial.

He examined the lymph glands which were enlarged near a skin cancer and found them choked with skin cells

—the cancerous cells—and through these glands the cells were spreading to other organs, the seeds of secondary cancer which are so difficult to eradicate. He also showed how cells acted in the repairing process. In the case of a wound, for instance, he showed that the bridging of the gap is achieved by the cells splitting off from the tissue around.

This work of Virchow's made the disease processes intelligible. However irrational the behavior of a disease there was a rational explanation. "All cells," declared Virchow, "come from other cells."

4. THE GLAND ORCHESTRA

Virchow's work was the beginning of the closer researches into the nature and structure of the organs of the body. This in turn was finally to dispose of the Salernan "humors" by the later discoveries of the endocrine, or ductless, glands.

There are the body glands, or organs, like the spleen, which produce chemicals which they supply to the blood or to the digestive system through ducts or tubes. But there are other glands which do not have ducts. The blood vessels run through them and absorb the chemicals directly.

These are the most significant glands in the body because they control not only our temperaments but the functions of the body and, indeed, of the emotions. They produce what are called "hormones" from a Greek word meaning "to excite," but some of them act as inhibitors, as depressors and not as exciters. Perhaps a better description of them would be "chemical messengers." These "messengers" are sent out, like minute men, through the blood stream, summoning, not only the organs of the body, but each other to instant action.

The anatomists of the seventeenth century were intrigued by what they called "the little brain," situated under the brain about midway between the top of the nose and the back of the skull. This we now know as the *pituitary,* or hypophysis. It is about the size of a green pea and consists of three parts—the anterior lobe, the posterior lobe, and an intermediate part, and it is situated immediately beneath the oldest part of the brain. Over this has been superimposed, by evolution, those parts of the brain which are concerned with the mind and the intellect. Scientists now know the hypophysis as the chemical laboratory which converts the telegraphic code of the brain into chemical "prescriptions" that are sent posthaste through the body.

It has also been called the "leader of the gland orchestra." For, with the subtle rhythm of the conductor who subdues the "strings" and summons the "brasses," the pituitary gland retards one gland while it stimulates another. Thus the gland system is kept in harmony. If each does not respond properly there is discord, which finds expression in disease.

Other ductless glands are the *pineal,* which is also situated in the brain and is also about the size of a pea; the *thyroid* gland in the neck; the *parathyroid,* adjoining the thyroid; the *thymus* gland in the chest; the *Islets of Langerhans,* on the pancreas; and *gonads,* or sex glands, which not only produce external secretions but also feed chemicals into the blood which produce the secondary sex characteristics; and the *adrenals,* capsules on the kidneys.

5. ORCHESTRA LEADER

The more the scientists examine the *pituitary* gland, or *hypophysis,* the more they are amazed at the complexity of the chemicals which are produced from this tiny body.

Overactivity of its anterior lobe during childhood results in *gigantism.* Such overactivity happening in adult life produces a condition known as *acromegaly,* the distressing effect of enlarging the extremities. The victims have large protruding jaws and noses, massive hands and feet, and as the disease progresses they die.

The hypophysis is associated with the growth of the body; with the regulation of the storage of fat. Excessive action leads to overgrowth and underactivity tends to produce a failure of the development of the skeleton accompanied by an increase in fatness. It also plays an important part in the control of the heartbeat and of the blood vessels. Injections of extracts of the gland stimulate the heart and increase the blood pressure. They also stimulate contractions of the intestines, of the bladder and of the womb, and are used to help childbirth.

The gland is also prominent in relation to the sex

glands and the sex impulses and in the processes of conception, pregnancy and birth. It is, in fact, the master organ of sex.

The hypophysis also has a part to play in the mechanism of sleep. Hibernation in animals is due to a lowering of the activity of this gland. First, there is the deep sleep; secondly, there is a fall in the bodily temperature—a condition associated with underactivity of the hypophysis; thirdly, there is the storage of fat, with the help of this gland, upon which the animal exists during his quiescent period. As the winter months approach, the pituitary prepares for the months during which the animal must live without external support by laying up a store of fat. With the onset of hibernation there is a regulated fall in temperature and a cessation of the bodily functions.

During normal sleep in a human being the same functions are in suspense. Digestion is at a standstill. Hence the ill effects which often ensue if a meal is eaten before going to bed.

It is a curious fact that sleep arrives periodically, no matter how the day has been spent. Observations of the surface of the brain during sleep have established the fact that there is a low blood supply, and that any increase in the blood to the brain during sleep is apt to disturb the sleeper. When the hypophysis is underactive, the usual rhythm of sleep is disturbed and the patient can drop off to sleep at any moment. This is in contrast to the normal person, who, when refreshed by sleep, has no desire for more. Also, the bodily temperature drops during sleep and there is diminished oxidation, so that less fat is burnt up. Fat people are much more somnolent than thin, and fat people are usually deficient in pituitary.

This gland is obviously a kind of clock and a calendar.

An example of its emotional relationship is found in the case of the cow who dislikes the milker and will not part with its milk. The farmer, in practice, would put the calf near the mother and the maternal emotion would release the milk against her will. An injection of extract of the hypophysis will make her do that, without the calf. It overrides her antagonisms and releases her emotions.

A well-developed anterior lobe of the hypophysis is often associated with imaginative force; the fortunate possessor is also often musical and a practical visionary. At the same time a slight deficiency in the pituitary may lead the person to try to compensate for his lack of the essential hormone by persistent conscientious effort, often in excess of his physical strength.

One of the ironies of our times is that the movies have glorified the "vital statistics" of female stars. The most prominent of these "statistics"—the pneumatic bustiness of women—can often be clinically identified as due to a defect of the pituitary, emphasizing the mammary glands.

6. *THE EYE OF CYCLOPS*

The *pineal* body was regarded by Descartes (1596-1650) as "the seat of the soul." Others regarded it as the "Eye of Cyclops" and maintained it to be the survival of a third eye. Its functions are still imperfectly understood, although it appears to attain its highest development in children, and tumors of the pineal body have been known to produce sexual precocity even in children of five years of age. It may have some association with the cross-over from childhood to young manhood which takes place at puberty.

7. *THE PACEMAKER*

The *thyroid* receives its name on account of its proximity to a shield-shaped cartilage in the throat—"thyroid" is from the Greek word meaning "a shield." As a rule the gland can be seen as an indefinite swelling on either side of what is known as the "Adam's apple" in the throat. The average weight of the gland is about an ounce but it weighs a little more in the female than in the male and enlarges during pregnancy. This gland is very much involved with the emotions. Anyone with an overfunctioning thyroid (like the poet, Shelley) has difficulty with the restrictions which society imposes and is irritable and explosive and may gradually develop actual insanity with suicidal tendencies.

Enlargements of the gland, caused by a deficiency of iodine in the diet, produce what is called goiter. This was one of the reasons for the original study of the thyroid. After the introduction of antiseptic surgery the surgeons in Switzerland, where goiter is common, were encouraged to remove the unsightly swellings, but when they did so their patients exhibited very distressing symptoms. They became slow in their muscular and intellectual responses, their features coarsened, and their hair became dry and fell out. If they were young, all further growth was arested and there was produced what we know as a *cretin*. This condition has been met nowadays by iodine therapy, and in recent years where malignant growths occur in the thyroid, by the use of radioactive isotopes. A natural cretin, given injections of extracts of the thyroid gland, can be restored and become a normal being.

3. SKELETON KEY

The *parathyroid* glands, usually four in number, are situated in close relation to the thyroid and at one time were supposed to be part of it. These glands are also concerned with growth but mainly, perhaps, in the building of the skeleton, since they are associated with calcium metabolism, the use of lime salts in the body. When the glands are removed from animals, tetany results. This disorder involves convulsions, shivering, and eventually death, and is also found in cases of deficiency of vitamin D, which plays a part in the calcium metabolism and the growth of teeth and bones; and it can also be produced by an excess of alkaline salts. A powerful extract has been obtained from the parathyroid, which can immediately remove the symptoms of tetany.

4. EMOTION BUFFER

The *thymus* is a curious gland in the chest, which is apparently not indispensable to life because people survive after its removal and there has been no noticeable change in the general metabolism, muscular strength or intelligence, nor does the operation appear to react on the other ductless glands. But it is believed that this is a dominant gland of childhood since it diminishes after puberty—shrinks as the activity of the sex organs increase. It has been found that the thymus is enlarged in adult eunuchs. It appears to have a restraining action on sexual development and where it persists unimpaired in adult life, it affects the sexual behavior and character, and may explain abnormal tendencies which are generally regarded as the province of the psychologist, rather than the physiologist.

A child with an abnormal thymus is the "angel child," delicate and fragile, like a piece of Dresden china. In the grown person with a persistent thymus, there is a large man with a smooth, hairless and fleshy face. The influence of the thymus is more marked in men than in women and it has been suggested that this gland may have a relationship to the male sex organs as the thyroid has to the female—although the glands are neither exclusively feminine or masculine.

Recent researches seem to suggest that the thymus is somehow a "buffer" gland, because, when animals are subjected to severe shock, the post-mortem examination shows that the gland has shriveled, like a pricked air cushion.

10. SUGAR CONTROLLER

One of the spectacular successes of gland therapy is the use of insulin in the treatment of diabetes. This insulin is the hormone from the *Islets of Langerhans*. In 1889 Mehring and Minkowski of Germany demonstrated that the removal of the pancreas resulted in diabetes. The experiments proved that in the absence of this gland, and more particularly in the absence of the portion of the pancreas which contains a little cluster of cells known as the Islets of Langerhans, diabetes occurred.

The *external* secretion of the pancreas is discharged into the top part of the small intestine. It is a pale yellow fluid and contains ferments which help to digest the food as it passes through the stomach.

The *internal* secretion, however, comes from these Islets and controls the amount of sugar in the blood. If the amount of sugar is excessive the victim will ultimately die of toxins that will form in the blood; if it is insufficient he will collapse into unconsciousness or a coma, which may be fatal.

Diabetes has been common throughout the ages but is even more common today because, as happens in the interaction between the glands and the nervous system, it can be caused by great nervous strain. In America there is a saying: "When the stock prices fall, diabetes rises." It has been shown experimentally that students under the nerve strain of a university examination will produce the evidence of diabetes.

In certain fish the glands are not scattered in the pancreas but form a separate gland of considerable size. At the beginning of this century, Rennie and Fraser, of Aberdeen University, studying fish which they got in the fish market of Aberdeen, considered the possible benefit of feeding these glands to diabetic patients. The treatment was without success because the digestive juices destroyed the protein of which insulin is composed. Therefore, it never reached the blood system which was crying out for it. The scientists realized this and tried the effect of injecting a watery extract of the gland under the skin. They were within reach of the discovery of insulin then, but, unfortunately, the extract was impure and set up an irritation which made it impossible for the patients to continue.

In Aberdeen at that time was J. J. R. Macleod, who was later to become a professor at Toronto University, where, in 1921, one of his colleagues, Dr. Frederick Banting, discussed with him the possibility of securing an extract from the Islets after causing the remaining secreting portion of the pancreas to degenerate by tying the ducts. Remembering the efforts of Rennie and Fraser, Macleod encouraged him to go ahead with the experiments, and Banting, with his colleague Charles Best, worked for months using extracts from the concentrated insulin in the tied-up pancreas to inject into diabetic dogs.

It was found that some of the dogs after receiving a strong extract would die, usually overnight. This was when they were not under observation and when they were not given a starchy meal to produce emergency sugar to counteract the effects of an overdose of insulin. A careful adjustment of the dosage was, therefore, necessary, and eventually a highly purified form of the hormone was obtained.

Insulin, vastly improved in its action since those days, is now plentiful and available and keeps patients alive without the miseries and wastage of the disease. A diabetic on an insulin regimen can lead a practically normal life. The insulin, however, is not a cure for diabetes. It merely holds the disease in check and the patients can live a normal life only as long as they can use it. But any lapse may bring sudden death.

There can be no cure for diabetes, since, in the advanced diabetic, the chemical factory, the glands which produce the insulin in the body, have closed down and the supplies must, therefore, come by injection from outside.

11. LOVE GLANDS

The term *gonad,* from the Greek word meaning "seed," is applied to any of the gamete-producing organs and includes what is meant by "sex glands." When we use the term it usually implies the means of reproduction. But a great deal more is involved in the sex glands than the secretions necessary for the reproduction of the species.

The glands also produce internal secretions which have a great deal to do with the physical, emotional, and temperamental characteristics of the two sexes. While the "primary" sexual differences are recognizable from birth, what are called "secondary sexual characteristics" make their appearance at puberty. It is then that the boy becomes a young man and the girl develops those changes in mind and body with which everyone is familiar. These changes are due to the *internal* secretions of the gonads. If the gonads, male and female, are damaged or removed the characteristics of manhood and womanhood fail to develop. This shows that a stimulant to the body chemistry has been removed.

In the case of the removal of the gonads in the female the general bodily shape gradually takes on male characteristics, while experiments have shown that the inplantation of female gonads into a young male animal results in a modification of his physical characteristics and behavior. But experimental grafting of the male gland into young female animals produces physical changes veering towards male characteristics and accompanied by a typical active pugnacity. Similarly the injection of the male or female hormone in the opposite sex produces recognizable changes.

The functions of the sex glands in man are more easily understandable than they are in woman. In the case of the female the sex instinct is complicated by the maternal instinct, which is a more widespread impulse and more complex in its effects.

The sex glands are very much part of the "gland orchestra," and sexual desire is bound up with the pituitary and thyroid glands. The relation with the thymus has already been mentioned but there are also involved the adrenals, which we are about to discuss, and which have been described as those responsible for distinctive masculinity. But this is probably exemplified mainly in pugnacity, which, of course, in the case of the male animal is most violent at the time of sexual impulse; then the male animals will violently fight one another for the females. While the thyroid gland appears to be particularly involved in the emotional life of women, the pituitary also plays a very large part in the female internal economy; it is involved in the menstrual cycle, in the processes of conception and pregnancy and birth, and in the suckling of the infant.

At the critical periods of change, the interplay of the sex hormones with the other glands produces the physical differentiations and changes, as at puberty and the climacteric, and, as is well known, these are periods of emotional disturbance.

12. SEX APPEAL

What is called "sex" in terms of the movies and the romantic novels—with its overtones of "sex-appeal" and male aggressiveness—is a cacophony of the "gland orchestra" in which the sex glands as such play an important but incidental part. In animals, the sex play is instinctive. In human beings, the stimulus is largely psychological and the impulses from the higher cortical centers of the brain, the thinking part, are communicated to the glandular system, which in turn reacts on the mental processes, creating mental or "romantic" stimulation. This action and reaction of mind and glands is, as the psychiatrists' engagement books testify, an increasing complication in our modern society. But the psychiatrists are coping with the end-result of a process which involves also the endocrinologists and the neurologists, who deal with the chemistry and the nervous energy of the body.

"Love" and "infatuation" have very little to do with the question of marriage and reproduction in primitive communities. Arranged marriages in which the parties have little choice; or propinquity marriages—neighborhood assessment of the marital qualities of a man or a woman—replace what we in advanced societies regard as romance. Perhaps this advance, away from animal instincts, is a higher attribute, but what appears to be discrimination in choice is itself indiscriminate in terms of the processes of reproduction. The decline in fertility in highly developed communities, as well as unhappy and broken marriages, has a great deal to do with the secretions of the sex glands, both external and internal.

As Francis Galton (1822-1911), a cousin of Charles Darwin, who was one of the first to study heredity experimentally, pointed out: wealthy heiresses, who generally come from infertile families with no brothers and few sisters to share the fortune, inherit also a low fertility. The dying-off of noble families can be traced to the fact that, to get the wealth to ensure their lineage, they married infertile heiresses, and curtailed it.

Just as, among birds and insects, coloration is a guide to the selection of mates, so among humans coloration is usually a guide to the endocrine secretions of the subject. Outward appearances give hints as to the endocrine personality—a measure of the relative functioning of the glands. Size, hair, eyes, complexion, relative length of the extremities and the trunk, all show endocrine values. Prescribers of medicine are taught that blondes require larger dosage than brunettes and that Indians, and the dark and yellow races in general, react to smaller doses than those which white people require. This probably means that the lighter races are more resistant to the action of chemicals by virtue of their pituitary domination.

What happens, therefore, when a man whose endocrines tell him that he ought to marry a blonde finds himself married to a bleached brunette? What happens when the upstate boy who would have married the mousy girl next door and would have found her glandularly compatible, becomes infatuated by the girl behind the cigar counter, a passionate Spanish type with an overactive postpituitary? Sociologists, concerned about the instability of human relationships, ought to get together with the endocrinologists.

13. FIGHT OR FLIGHT

The *adrenals* have been left to the end of this recital of the glands because of the new significance which they have begun to acquire.

Adrenalin was the first of the active principles of the endocrine glands to be obtained in crystalline form, by

Jokichi Takamine in 1901. This came from the *medulla* or core of the adrenal, or suprarenal, glands, which are capsules on the top of each of the kidneys.

Adrenalin is the chemical hormone of *fight* or *flight,* being the chemical that causes the body to react to the stimulus of fright or fear. If a person is startled by the appearance of an enemy the adrenalin will either help him to punch him in the jaw or help him to run away. The hormone diffuses rapidly through the sympathetic nervous system and acts on the various organs and muscles; the heart beats faster; the spleen contracts and increases the amount of blood circulating; the lungs are relaxed; and the liver gives out more sugar, necessary for the energy of muscle action. The pupil of the eye dilates and the eyeball protrudes—"pops out of the head." The chemical acts on the intestine—"fear gripping the stomach." The vessels of the skin are constricted, producing "gooseflesh," and the hairs stand erect from the contraction of the muscles of the skin. This last can be seen in the rising hackles of a frightened dog or the fur standing up on a cat whose body muscles have contracted to arch its back. This would seem to be one of the "tricks" of nature to make an animal look bigger in the presence of threat.

The action of adrenalin is apparent in everyday situations. If a person is crossing the road and is startled by the hooter of an approaching car, he will react. He cannot stand and *fight* the car, therefore the instinct is *flight.* With a leap or a sprint of which he would probably be incapable in ordinary circumstances he will dodge out of the way and stand on the sidewalk with his heart thumping, his lungs panting and a weak feeling in his abdomen. He will feel dizzy and have a bursting feeling in the head and may actually be physically sick. It is known that the adrenal *medulla* produces these effects because they can be reproduced by injections of the crystalline adrenalin.

One of the beneficial effects of this hormone is that it can be used in cases where the patient's heart has stopped beating on the operating table. It can have the effect of jerking the heart back into motion.

So much for the *medulla.* Over this core there is a *cortex* or "bark." This "bark" has been intensively engaging the interest of research scientists.

It produces and secretes no fewer than twenty-eight

different chemicals, including some very powerful ones. A disturbance of the adrenal cortex by a tumor or by wastage can produce a "change" of sex even in a grown person. The bearded woman of the circus is an example of adrenal dysfunction. But a tumor on the adrenal of a woman may produce even more extraordinary effects than that. A woman will find to her horror that she is progressively changing her sex. She feels as Jekyll felt in becoming Hyde. She begins to grow masculine hair and her voice begins to deepen, her sexual behavior changes and in some cases the sexual organs themselves may be modified so that the victim becomes a case, which the tabloids love, of the woman who becomes the bridegroom of a woman.

Then there is *cortisone,* a product of the adrenal *cortex*. This was the sensation of 1949. Here was the drug which was going to cure rheumatoid arthritis, that disease which cripples millions—seven million in the United States and two million in Britain.

For its discovery Dr. Philip S. Hench and Dr. Edward Kendall, of the Mayo Clinic, and Professor T. Reichstein, the Swiss, were awarded the Nobel Prize in 1950.

Dr. Hench, twenty years before, had noticed that men and women with arthritis had less pain when they had jaundice; that women expecting babies often had their rheumatism relieved; and that rheumatic patients who had surgical operations for other reasons, were temporarily benefited. Here was a piece of acute scientific observation. There must be something more than a coincidence in the three very different circumstances.

The scientists speculated whether in the adrenal cortex there might not be yet another substance, which they called "Substance X," which would prove to be the antirheumatic factor. They were looking to the adrenal because the secretions of the cortex are particularly active in jaundice, in childbirth, and in the response of the body to surgical operations.

After years of biochemical research, Compound E was extracted from the adrenal glands of cattle. It could also be extracted from bile, which provided the link with jaundice. In 1949, the first cases were treated and the results were dramatic enough to make the headlines. Patients who had been completely bedridden, with crippled joints and unable to move, let alone walk, were out of bed within a few days. Within a week, under treatment, pain and muscular stiffness had disappeared and the patients could literally dance a jig with relief. But it was not a "cure," any more than insulin is a "cure" for diabetes, and, like diabetes, rheumatism could only be kept in hand as long as regular injections of Compound E were given. As soon as the injections stopped, the patients relapsed into their previous condition, the more miserable in fact because of the temporary well-being they had experienced.

It was then found that similar effects could be obtained by means of another hormone, ACTH, or Adreno-Cortico-Tropic Hormone, obtained from the anterior lobe of the pituitary, or hypophysis, gland, which controls the adrenals. Remove it, and the glands on the kidneys shrivel. Restore it by transplantation or by injections of ACTH, and the adrenals function again. In rheumatic cases, ACTH encouraged the adrenals to produce the deficient cortisone.

Cortisone, as far as the rheumatoid arthritis is concerned, has not lived up to the promises of the headlines. It has what are called "side effects," which is understandable in terms of the known relationship of the cortex to the sex-system. Women treated with cortisone for the long periods necessary to maintain respite from rheumatoid arthritis, begin to develop beards and mustaches and male characteristics. But there are other dangers. Patients may become more susceptible to infections—if tuberculosis, for instance, is latent it may flare up.

These considerations, although they may be disappointing to the high hopes of rheumatism sufferers, do not alter the fact that cortisone was a great discovery. To the scientists, the puzzling effects only make it the more interesting.

That is the difference between the scientific approach to medicine and the trial-and-error methods by which experience of drugs was built up in the past. Physicians in the old days would not persist with the drug if they found it had ill effects as well as beneficial ones. The biochemist today is not put off; he asks why? The result of the discovery of and disputation about cortisone stimulated intense investigations of the hormones of the cortex and their action. This has produced a newer concept of the human body.

14. REVOLT IN THE BODY STATE

Virchow said: "The body is a cell-state in which every cell is a citizen. Disease is merely a conflict of the citizens of the state brought about by the action of external forces."

This "action of external forces" obviously would be true of germ diseases, invading from outside, and nutritional diseases due to deficiencies in the food from outside. But how could it apply to the internal economy of the body state? How could it apply to the degenerative diseases like thickening of the arteries, weakening of the heart, increasing of the blood pressure, failure of the glands (as in diabetes) and to cancerous growths, etc?

In general, these could be described as gross manifestations of the normal processes of aging—the wearing out of the machinery of the body. But, of course, these diseases are not confined to the older age groups and their increasing appearance in younger age groups is a matter of deep concern in the highly developed societies. From the evidence of what happens among one's own friends one must conclude that the stress and strain of modern life is having an effect.

This is obvious from the statistics of the World Health Organization. We can roughly classify diseases as *mass diseases, degenerative diseases* and *stress diseases*. The first classification applies to those diseases which are so widespread in a country and affect so high a proportion of the population as to be a dominant factor in hindering social and economic development and which, medically, mask other diseases to the point of making them clinically irrelevant until the *mass diseases* are removed. These are the infectious and communicable diseases. Malnutrition would come in the same category. When these mass diseases are brought under control "new" diseases such as polio appear to emerge. Of course, they are not new. They have existed previously but have been masked or inhibited by the mass diseases.

As has been said, the *degenerative* diseases are those which are associated normally with older age groups—diseases of the heart and circulation, brain hemorrhages, organic and glandular disorders and cancers. More than half the people who die in the eight countries which have the highest per capita income die from diseases of the heart and circulation systems and from cancers.

Stress diseases include gastric and duodenal ulcers, diabetes and nervous breakdowns, as well as the appearance of the degenerative diseases in younger age groups.

Today if one correlates these classifications to countries, one finds that mass diseases apply to the underdeveloped countries, degenerative diseases to countries with a rising standard of life, and stress diseases to highly developed countries where the tempo of life has changed and where people live at a high speed, under insistent economic and emotional pressures.

Every person is subject to the conditions of the world in which he or she lives and the stresses which it imposes. Dr. Hans Selye, director of the University of Montreal's Institute of Experimental Medicine and Surgery, provoked world-wide interest and (as always) medical dispute by his experiments to show that all disease is a result of something which impinges on the body from outside and thus upsets the internal balance—Virchow's "action of external forces." He subjected experimental animals to the kind of assaults which human beings must endure. He subjected them to bitter cold and intense heat. He starved them, frightened them, and shocked them. A post-mortem examination showed that whatever the cause of death may have been, the adrenal glands were always swollen and discolored, the thymus gland had shriveled, and the stomach was ulcerated. There was thus a common factor, which Selye called "the stress factor."

Studies of the blood and body fluids have shown that as soon as any animal is subjected to stress there is an "alarm reaction." It is like the scream of an air-raid siren which mobilizes Civil Defense. In the same way the body mobilizes its defenses. The command post is apparently the adrenal cortex. It injects hormones into the blood stream and immediately they pervade the whole body. The hormones "trim" the body for the crisis by adjusting its water and salt content and by raising the amount of sugar in the blood, to provide the energy for the emergency. But the adrenals do this at the command of the pituitary, or hypophysis, itself reacting to the mental stimuli. If the pituitary is removed there is no alarm reaction. If the adrenals are removed there is no adequate defense system.

Just as a Civil Defense organization becomes exhausted by repeated air-raids, so does the defense system of the body. In the first instance the alarm reaction produces the proper changes in the tissues and organs. This is called "the stage of resistance." Having thus adapted itself, and the crisis having passed, the body returns to normal. But if the onset has been severe or the alarms repeated too often the subject may die of cold or fright. This is "the stage of exhaustion."

In experimental animals subjected to stress, one finds a thickening of the arteries, high blood pressure, heart disease and stomach ulcers. Selye's suggestion was that the adrenals were being overzealous. In a desperate attempt to meet the stress they were pouring out hormones in too large amounts.

The effects can be understood when we consider the contradictions which occur when cortisone or ACTH is administered. If a person has gout either hormone will relieve it, but if either is given to a patient subject to gout at a time when it is quiescent, it will cause the gout to flare up. The hormones appear to check tuberculosis, but again they are liable to cause latent tuberculosis to become active. They appear at first to relieve high blood pressure, but again the relief is only temporary.

It is obvious from this, and other studies of the endocrines, that the normal body is in a state of delicate balance which external influences can profoundly disturb.

The mind, the nervous system and the glands all react to emotional disturbances and interact one upon the other to produce not only temperamental but physical changes. The Tired Business Man, with four telephones going at once, is not only under the stress of making judgments; his nerves are "jangled" and his endocrines are "spluttering." Result: stomach ulcers, or prematurely hardened arteries or a heart attack.

In an age of specialization in which medical experts begin to know more and more about their specific specialty, the stress diseases ought to be a reminder of The Whole Man—the inseparable relationship of mind and body.

This interplay of the mental processes on the body organs and of the organs on the mind is what is referred to by the word "psychosomatic."

Part Eight.

THE GREAT ADVANCES (V)

> It is not without significance that in The
> Lord's Prayer, the petition for our daily
> bread has priority even over the petition
> for the forgiveness of sins, a fact worthy
> of consideration by The Churches . . . .
>
> —LORD BOYD-ORR: *The White Man's
> Dilemma*

1. SCOTT OF THE ANTARCTIC

"Good-bye—I am not at all afraid of the end but sad to
miss many a simple pleasure which I had planned for the
future in our long marches. . . . We are in a desperate
state—feet frozen, etc., no fuel and a long way from
food, but it would do your heart good to be in our tent
and to hear our cheery conversation. . . . We are very
near the end. . . . We did intend to finish ourselves when
things proved like this but we have decided to die naturally. . . ."

That was the penciled note which was found beside
the bodies of Captain Robert Falcon Scott and his companions in the tent in which they died after losing the race
to the South Pole to Amundsen. It was addressed to J. M.
Barrie, the author, and I can remember strong men sob-
bing as Barrie read it aloud for the first time.

Wherever men talk of heroes and high courage, the
names of Robert Falcon Scott and that "very gallant
gentleman," Lawrence (Titus) Oates, are hailed and hallowed—Scott, accepting death as he had accepted defeat,
and Oates, walking out into the Antarctic blizzard to die,
lest he be a burden to his companions.

*Yet they need not have died. Scott's Southern Party did
not starve to death. They died of lack of Vitamin C.*

Sir Raymond Priestley, who had been a member of
the Scott Expedition at the age of twenty-three, said in
his presidential address to the British Association in 1956:

"The weather was unkind. Nevertheless scurvy was

151

the decisive factor. Under man-hauling conditions four
months is about as long as men hauling sledges can live
on rations completely devoid of Vitamin C. Once that
period elapsed, nervous and physical deterioration were
bound to set in, sores would refuse to heal and lassitude
would supervene."

Indeed that is the litany of Vitamin C deficiency. There
is a saying in the East:

> Better to walk than to run;
> Better to sit than to walk;
> Better to sleep than to sit;
> Better to die than to wake.

It is true that when Scott made his South Pole dash
in 1912 we were still a long way from knowing the A-Z
of vitamins (and we still are), but the reader will remember Wendell Holmes's "Medicine learned from a
sailor how to keep off scurvy," and the account (in Part
One) of how the Royal Navy (of which Scott was an officer) had made lemon juice compulsory, as an anti-
scurvy precaution, on all voyages. Strange, therefore, that
Scott should have overlooked this necessity. But, as Raymond Priestley said of his dead leader, "He more than
atoned by the manner of his death."

Since those days, vitamins have become not only a
science but a cult. Vitamin therapy is no longer just the
prescription of a doctor who has diagnosed some deficiency. Supplementary vitamins are added to our food.
We take "vitamin cocktails" in the form of multiple-
vitamin pills "just in case." In summer, when nature is
lush in its supply of vitamins—plenty of sunlight to promote Vitamin D and enrich the Vitamin A foods and
plenty of fresh vegetables to supply Vitamin C and so on
—we still supercharge ourselves with synthetic vitamins.
Yet, as we have seen in our discussion of the chemistry of
the body, the chemical system of the body is discreet
and economical in its use of fine chemicals. Just as it
needs, and cannot function without, trace minerals, it
will rebel against metallic poisoning in excessive
amounts. So, too, with vitamins. There is such a thing as
"hypervitaminosis"—ill-effects from excessive vitamins.

As Sir Frederick Gowland Hopkins, the Nobel Prize
winner, and pioneer of vitamins once said to me in his

wise old age: "All that I have ever learned about vitamins has taught me what I don't know about vitamins. A vitamin is a unit by which we should measure our ignorance. Every new food-factor which is discovered is a reminder of those which we haven't discovered."

He spoke from his own experience, because he was recalling the arrogance of nineteenth-century science which he himself had broken down. He was recalling Justus von Liebig (1803-73) and what Hopkins called his "lusty self-confidence."

2. MAN, THE MACHINE

Liebig made four important contributions to the evolution of chemistry: First, he devised methods of analyzing organic matter. Secondly, he introduced the far-reaching idea of "compound radicals," which are compound groups of atoms which undergo many different chemical combinations but which, through every change, maintain their identity as a group. Thirdly, he first prepared many entirely new substances, including chloral and chloroform. Fourthly, he spent thirty years of his life investigating how the body employs the food which it consumes.

He divided foodstuffs into two classes, those which are used to supply energy and those which go to the building up of new tissues and to the repair of wear and tear. The first (*respiratory foods,* he called them) consist of the *carbohydrates,* sugars and fats; and the second are the *proteins,* or nitrogen-containing foods. His name is associated with the first artificial fertilizer and the first patent food. He had set down to his own satisfaction, and that of those who accepted his dogma, the essentials of food. How wrong he was! He had found just one or two clues to the cross-word puzzle and many more were to try (and are still trying) to fill in the squares. The answers could not lie only with the chemist.

Some of the clues lay with James Prescott Joule (1817-99), a brewer's son, who at the age of twenty-six read a paper at the British Association and read it very badly. It had the uninspiring title of *The Calorific Effects of Magnetic Electricity and the Mechanical Value of Heat,* and his audience was frankly bored until another young man of twenty-three bounced up in excitement and cried "A great truth and a great discovery!" He was William Thomson, later to become Lord Kelvin and, among many other things, to play a principal part in linking Europe and America by cable. But for that flash of insight on that young man's part, "Joule's Law" might have faded on the paper on which the lecture was written.

In Berlin, Hermann von Helmholtz (1821-94) was outraging his elders and betters by his brash interference with accepted ideas. At the age of twenty-six, while studying to become an army surgeon, he wrote an essay on the conservation of energy—and argued that all modes of energy, e.g., mechanical heat, light, electricity, sound, and all chemical phenomena, including those of the body, are capable of transformation from one to another, but are otherwise indestructible and impossible of creation. And he gave universal application, embracing physiology, to the law which four years before Joule had applied to physical phenomena.

His contemporary at the University of Berlin was Emil du Bois Reymond (1818-96), a German of French extraction. At the age of twenty-six (notice how it was the age of young ideas) he showed that in the contracting muscle there is a change in the electric potential (shown dramatically in the modern electrocardiograph); thus electricity as well as heat was produced by the body. Heat and electricity were forms of physical energy and, physiologically, chemical activity thus produced both. This fitted Helmholtz's unifying theory.

Another contemporary, in time though not in place, was Claude Bernard (1813-78) a winegrower's son from the vineyards of St. Julien. He had gone to Paris as a dramatist with a five-act tragedy. A critic to whom he showed it made the cynical suggestion that he had better take up medicine and maybe some wealthy woman patient would play "sugar-mammy" to his play. Bernard took the advice literally. He never found his backer because he became fascinated by research. *Arthur de Bretagne,* his play, was produced fifty years later but only in book form, as a memorial to France's greatest physiologist.

Bernard was the founder of experimental medicine—the artificial production of disease, for the purposes of research. At the age of thirty, he injected cane sugar directly into the veins and found that it was discarded in the urine. He then treated the sugar with gastric juice and found that the body retained it. This was the beginning of his investigation of the glycogenic function of the liver—that is, the production of animal starch which the liver releases as dextrose sugar as the body requires it. Bernard thus proved the existence of an "internal secretion" (a term which he invented) which showed that the animal body could build up substances as well as break them down, and that the living processes were not, as the disciples of Liebig insisted, just the decomposition of chemicals absorbed as food. Furthermore, it opened up the way to the discovery of hormones. Indeed, Bernard produced diabetes experimentally. His work on the nerves and the muscles and the control of the blood vessels started a whole train of inquiries into the electrochemical functions of the body.

Thus we have a unifying principle—something that is always liable to be overlooked in these days of over-specialization—Liebig's animal heat; Joule's physical heat; Bernard's chemical interactions; Bois-Reymond's electric pulses, and Helmholtz's conservation of energy in which to encompass them all.

Here we have a century ago, the claims staked out for what we know nowadays as biochemistry, biophysics and endocrinology (the study of the ductless glands). The way was opened to the discovery of hormones, enzymes and vitamins.

The first hurdle was *metabolism*. Pettenkofer (1818-1901) and Voit (1831-1908) started with the first stage of nutrition; *anabolism*, the conversion of foodstuffs into tissue. They studied the second stage; *katabolism*, the breaking down of food and discarded tissue into waste. But what of *metabolism*, the intermediate process in which the body produced *energy* from sugar or fat? How much energy per pound? How much incidental heat? How to arrive at a unit of measurement?

Ludwig II, King of Bavaria, provided the researchers with their apparatus. It was a sealed chamber in which a living body, man or animal, could be enclosed. The amount of air going in was measured and controlled and the kind of air which came out could be measured and analyzed and so could the amount remaining in the cabinet. A thermometer measured the heat. They fed their subject on fat alone; on carbohydrate alone; or protein alone; or they starved him. They showed that the energy value of food could be calibrated in the physical unit of heat—the calorie—as every dieter knows today. Each food contributed a certain number of calories—carbohydrates (sugars and starches) predominating—and the body, in its various conditions, consumed so many calories according to the effort expended.

It was all delightfully simple. Remember this was the heyday of The Machines. Here was the living body behaving exactly like a factory. There was a furnace to be stoked—so much food for so much effort, like so much coal to get so many pounds pressure of steam. The nervous system was Morse's telegraph. The stomach and digestive system was the through-put, with an adequate sewage system. The blood circulation was the conveyor belt, carrying oxygen and chemicals to the tissues and carrying away the waste products to join the waste food in the garbage. Simple? Too simple to be true!

Although Karl Marx did not realize it, his proletarian revolution was nearly achieved by mechanics other than those he had in mind—the mechanics of a too-mechanical concept. The Upper Classes were in imminent danger of being wiped out. Liebig and his followers had given them the opportunity of discarding the vulgar wet nurses, who suckled the scions; instead they could have Balanced Bottles for Bouncing Babies. The chemists could suckle the infants of those who could afford it and could promise plump offspring. They were plump, all right, but they had "Barlow's disease," which is infantile scurvy. Today baby foods are replete with vitamins and accessories but in those days these were unknown.

3. THE MISSING PARTS

We have dealt with scurvy, the first vitamin deficiency disease to be treated before its exact cause was discovered. But let us have a look at some of the other vitamin diseases.

There was Christiaan Eijkman (1858-1930) and his "drunken" poultry. Eijkman had been sent out from Holland to the Dutch East Indies to investigate the ravages of beriberi and he was not satisfied with his colleagues' report, although he agreed with them that it was due to a germ. He stayed behind to isolate the germ.

One day he noticed some fowls in a Javanese hospital

yard staggering around with limp necks and drooping wings, and his trained scientific mind immediately associated their behavior with the human affliction of beriberi. This was the more plausible because he found that the fowls were fed on the leavings on the plates of beriberi patients. He began bacteriological tests to find the "germs" thus transferred.

But his experiments were rudely interrupted by an officious new superintendent who was shocked to find that the fowls were being given milled rice (albeit, the leavings of the patients). Milled rice, with the bran removed, was "superior" rice, too good for poultry. So the fowls were fed—in spite of Eijkman's protests—on unmilled rice, which was supposed to be unsuitable for human consumption.

If that superintendent had not been so officious, Eijkman would not now have his place in history. He had abandoned the experiment and then one day was passing the fowl run and noticed that they were perking up and a few days later they were normal. Could it be that the milling of the rice caused the beriberi? And so it proved.

He followed up this observation by examining the records of prisons in Java. In thirty-seven, *unpolished rice* was served and in only one was there a case of beriberi. In fifty-one prisons, *polished rice* was served and in *only one* of them had the prisoners escaped beriberi. Until 1906, he still clung to the idea that the disease was due to a germ—refusing to recognize that it was in fact due to the absence of a "germ"—not bacterial, but the "germ" of the rice which was discarded with the bran in milling.

In 1906, Sir Frederick Gowland Hopkins, as a result of his researches into food, pronounced: "No animal can live upon a mixture of pure protein, fat and carbohydrate, and even when the necessary inorganic material is carefully supplied, the animal still cannot flourish."

He pursued his experiments. He fed young rats upon an artificial food mixture containing caseinogen, starch, cane sugar, lard and organic salts. He purified these constituents and the rats died. He found that growth stopped even when they were eating as much as they required. To another series of animals—a "control group"—he gave, in addition to this basal diet, a tiny quantity of milk, so small as not to amount to anything in terms of carbohydrate, fat or protein. The animals prospered. The answer was a fractional, elusive "something" in the diet—proof enough to justify his 1912 pronouncement on *The Importance of Accessory Food Factors in Normal Dietaries,* which revolutionized the approach to nutrition and gave us "vitamins." The word itself ("vitamines" with an "e") was invented by the Polish scientist, Casimir Funk, who first successfully extracted the chemical factor in the rice polishings which prevented beriberi.

An alphabet of vitamins then emerged. At first it was assumed that there was a universal vitamin—a sort of catalyst—but it was soon obvious that the factor which prevented scurvy was not the same as that which prevented beriberi. And the study of neither produced any explanation of the "growth factor," the absence of which prevented Hopkins' rats from developing. That was found by McCollum and Davis, two American investigators, in 1915, and labeled "Fat-soluble A." It was present in milk fat, butter and egg yolk, but not in lard or olive oil. Not only did it assist growth but it prevented night blindness and eye infections. This became "Vitamin A." Funk's anti-beriberi factor became "Vitamin B" and the anti-scurvy factor "Vitamin C."

4. SHADOW SICKNESS

Rickets—that disease of sunless slums—was not at first associated with the "growth factor," but Edward Mellanby, one of Hopkins' students, began to examine the various diet deficiencies which produce rickets in puppies. He found that cod-liver oil and other animal fats known to contain Vitamin A protected his puppies against rickets, while vegetable oils did not. But it was not until 1922 that he established that the so-called Vitamin A consisted of two factors—one growth-promoting and the other rickets-preventing. The second was renamed "Vitamin D."

The effects of Vitamin D, however, can be produced by sunlight and ultraviolet rays. But how? The answer was found by Steenbock, of the University of Wisconsin, who showed that rickets could be prevented just as well by irradiating the animals' food as by irradiating the animals. Even more strange was the fact that if the animal cages were irradiated before the animals were put in the vitamin effect was still produced. This was outrageous—

like going back to mesmerism and "putting the 'fluence" on inanimate metal. Even when it was found that the rats were eating irradiated sawdust in the cage, the scientists were still unhappy and shuddered at the thought that science was being invaded by a mystical concept, like the *élan vital* or something!

To escape from this sinister cabala, the chemists started to take to pieces the anti-rickets foodstuffs and to irradiate each fraction separately. They finally came down to the "sterols," the waxy materials associated with fats, and particularly to cholesterol. Then they found that when cholesterol was highly purified it no longer reacted to ultraviolet light nor had the Vitamin D effect. What they sought must then be an "impurity." This was ultimately found to be "ergosterol," so-called because it is best found in ergot, the fungus on rye. Further breakdown led to the discovery by Bourdillon and his colleagues at the National Institute for Medical Research, London, of the final fraction in pure crystalline form, which they called "calciferol" (because Vitamin D promotes the proper use of calcium in the bones and teeth). This synthetic Vitamin D is so potent that a watch crystal can hold a day's supply for a million children to keep them safe from rickets.

5. SUN SICKNESS

Without exhaustively, or chronologically, pursuing all the vitamins—in the 1930s, vitamin research was as fashionable as nuclear research is today and almost as many papers were being published on them—we might consider Vitamin B.

First, Vitamin B was regarded as one vitamin—anti-beriberi. Then it was found that it could be effective against pellagra, which Italians once called *mal del sole,* "sun sickness." This affliction, which once ranked among the greatest killer diseases in the United States, was finally identified by Dr. Joseph Goldberger of the U.S. Public Health Service. He went and lived among the Negroes and poor whites of the Deep South, where it was most prevalent. He tackled the problem in two ways: he proved that it was not due to infection and then he investigated the diet of the sufferers.

He discovered that those who suffered from it were

living on a diet poorer than their neighbors, who escaped, apparently, by eating fresh meat, eggs and milk. He then selected two orphan asylums and a lunatic asylum, where pellagra was rife among the patients. He banished the disease by providing more meat, vegetables, eggs and milk—not only preventing the disease but curing those who had it.

The next move was more dramatic. A group of convicts in a Mississippi prison were offered free pardons if they would volunteer to endure a diet modeled on that of the poorer cotton workers. Eleven agreed, and by the end of five months five of them had skin disease typical of pellagra. Goldberger had now to prove that the disease was not communicable. To establish this he and fifteen associates inoculated themselves with blood, nose droppings, urine, feces and peeling skin from pellagra patients. Unpleasant, but convincing! Pellagra was not infective.

Goldberger narrowed the food factor down to Funk's Vitamin B but then found that not all foods containing it were effective and that some foods which were useful in preventing beriberi did not prevent pellagra. By elimation, he "sorted out" the factor—a new, but related, vitamin which became known as B_2 (or "Vit. G").

How complex "B" can be is shown by the fact that one of the momentous discoveries of our times is B_{12}.

6. BLOOD SICKNESS

Before 1925, anyone who had pernicious anemia was under death sentence. Pernicious anemia is due to a failure of the marrow of the bone—the blood factory of the body—to produce enough red blood cells. The blood-producing function of the marrow depends on a chemical produced in the stomach and this, in turn, depends on the subtle chemistry of the body. In 1925, a young Boston physician, George R. Minot, started from the not unreasonable assumption that anemia patients did not eat enough meat. He and his colleague, William P. Murphy, began to feed them with the most concentrated form of all protein, the liver. To make sure that no value was lost in cooking, they administered it in minced, raw form. It was a nauseating diet, but it worked. Pernicious anemia victims became well but stayed well only as long as they persisted with the diet. The disease ceased to be a killer but the diet was unpalatable. Scientists began to search for whatever it was in the raw liver which acted on the stomach, and, through its secretions, on the marrow.

In 1948, Dr. Lester Smith and his colleague, L. F. J. Parker, of the Glaxo Laboratories, near London, set out to discover the ultimate factor. They used chromotography. This is a simple but ingenious idea, which is best demonstrated by dropping some ink on a blotter and watching it diffuse: it will spread out in a series of "haloes" of lighter and different shades; the chemical fractions in the ink are separating out. With more scientific precision, you can sort out the constituents of a chemical compound. In this case, the adsorbent was silica packed into a glass column, but the principle was the same as that of the blotting paper. The chemical compound—a known anti-anemia substance extracted from the liver—was poured in at the top and diffused through the adsorbent. Since the various fractions in the compound were adsorbed at a different rate, they began to separate out and appeared as varicolored stripes, horizontally across the pillar.

A thin red cross section which appeared in the adsorbent "candle" was cut out and examined. It was the factor for which they were looking. When tried on patients it was highly effective—thousands of times more potent than any other treatment for pernicious anemia. Then they managed to crystallize it—the first step toward synthesis. They began extensive clinical trials in hospitals.

Meanwhile, an American team, in the Merck laboratories, were after the same thing and arrived at the same result but they also found a quicker way of testing it than by clinical trials on human patients. Dr. Mary Shore of Maryland University had found that a germ culture of *Lactobacillus,* the bacterium which sours milk, reacted in measurable terms to the pernicious anemia factor; so the American discovery was tried on that and all the necessary confirmation was obtained. The American announcement appeared in the U.S. journal *Science* before Lester Smith's pronouncement was made.

The factor was called "Vitamin B_{12}" and was a phenomenal discovery, not only because of its beneficial effect but because it was the most powerful biological chemical known to man—a millionth of a gram can restore the red blood cells in normal circulation. It does not "cure," since it is a substitute, like insulin, for something which is permanently lacking in the body.

It is now known that Vitamin B_{12} is not produced in the liver. It is produced by fermentation by micro-organisms, and its main source for manufacturing purposes nowadays is the molds which produce antibiotic drugs. One of the aspects of pernicious anemia which baffled experts when it was supposed to be a by-product of liver had been: How did non-meat-eating herbivorous creatures obtain their supplies? The answer now became clear: by fermentation in the rumen. Humans obtained it from their food, but only if the so-called "intrinsic factor" in the gastric glands was present to select it and feed it to the liver to store for blood-forming purposes. It is the "intrinsic factor" which is lacking in pernicious anemia patients, and injection of B_{12} into the blood overcomes the defect.

7. RADIOACTIVE DRUGS

How does a substance like Vitamin B_{12} go to work inside the body? Obviously, its behavior is too subtle for direct observation (like Beaumont's window into St. Martin's stomach), and, since it is a living substance, there is no way of studying it in the dissecting room. But, nowadays, the biochemists have been given powerful new tools in the radioactive isotopes, elements which are the by-products of atomic energy.

A radioactive isotope is the "twin" of the ordinary element. Although it gives off radiations, it will behave chemically like its natural "twin," form the same chemical compounds, follow the same processes, and go, in the body, wherever the other would have gone. Lester Smith and his colleague Dr. D. R. Mallin, of the Post-Graduate Medical School, London, took Vitamin B_{12}, now identified as the chemical compound *cyanocobalt-amin*, which, as the name indicates, includes the element, cobalt. They replaced, by tricks the modern chemists have learned, the ordinary cobalt by its radioactive twin. Thus they were able to trace the vitamin through the body processes. They were able to study how it was absorbed in a curative way but they also used the vitamin as a research instrument to discover the nature of the disease process of pernicious anemia.

At the United Nations Conference on the Peaceful Uses of Atomic Energy at Geneva in 1955, medical scientists from all countries came along with their evidence of how in the hitherto mysterious recesses of the human body the labeled atoms can report back information. Just as they can discover how Vitamin B_{12} encourages blood-cell production, so they can find what elements are selectively filtered through the membranes of the blood vessels, and how the various elements travel to their destination—calcium to the bone, for instance, or iodine to the thyroid.

And if you know you can convert your researches into treatment. Radioactive iodine, rapidly concentrated in the thyroid, can be used as a treatment for the disorders of that gland. Radiophosphorus can be used as a means of controlling *leukemia,* the overproduction of white cells in the blood, or *polycythemia vera,* the overproduction of red blood cells. Radioactive gold can be injected straight into a tumor or into a cavity where the seeds of cancer may be gathering. Or boron may be injected into the veins, and will find its way to the brain and concentrate in a tumor if it exists. The boron itself is not radioactive but if it is bombarded by a beam of neutrons it will give off intense rays which attack the tumor without affecting the other parts of the brain.

Although penicillin "worked" in its prevention of the multiplication of germs, no one knew how until it was "labeled." Radioactive atoms were "tacked on" by adding them to the nutrient which feeds the mold, which produces the penicillin. It was found that the penicillin did not penetrate the germ sufficiently to kill it, but apparently it alters the chemicals on which the germ depends for its survival and propagation.

8. RADIOACTIVE MOSQUITOES

Radioactive tabs are used to study the behavior of germs themselves, and the ways in which disease is communicated.

One of the first lines of attack is on the carriers of disease, from the housefly, which can be branded with isotopes and tracked, to the viruses, which can be labeled and studied in transmission. Flies can be made to pick up radioactive filth and can be followed—sometimes as far as thirty miles. In this way the scientists can make a detailed survey of the habits of flies—an important factor in relation to the spread of dysentery and polio. Similarly, ticks, mites, fleas, lice and other "hosts" of disease can be made to disclose the methods of communicating disease to man. The influenza virus, the plague bacillus and the tuberculosis bacterium have all been labeled and tracked.

Arctic flowers were made radioactive, by feeding them with radioactive fertilizer, and the mosquitoes sipping their nectar picked up the tracers and thereafter became marked, and emitted rays. They were like a fugitive criminal who had stolen a working transmitter—the detectives with a receiver (or the mosquito-chasing entomologists with a Geiger counter) could follow him to any hide-out.

Pollens can be labeled in the same way so that we might find out how they cause allergies, like hay fever.

That ancient and intractable disease, leprosy, can now be cured by the use of basic sulfone drugs, but the results are inconstant. The mechanism by which the disease spreads through the body, as well as the action of the drug in human patients, can be accurately assessed if labeled atoms are used.

Thus the atom presents immeasurable possibilities in research, in diagnosis, in prevention and in treatment of the ails which afflict the human body.

9. FROM THE SUN TO THE CELL

But radioactive isotopes can also provide information of a much wider significance—something which reinforces Helmholtz's "unity," the conservation of energy, encompassing mechanical heat, light, sound, electricity and all chemical phenomena as forms of energy.

The source of all life on earth is the sun, but how does the sun's energy, intangible rays, become the food we eat, and the vitamins, hormones and cells? An essential stage in the process is *photosynthesis*, by which the growing plant traps the energy from the sun and uses it to compound the elements from the air, soil and water, into the food we eat.

The key lies in *chlorophyll*, the green substance which

traps the sun's rays and resembles in its method of synthesis the formation of blood cells in animals.

Gradually, scientists using labeled atoms have been drawing blueprints of the plant's chemical laboratory. Dr. Melvin Calvin, of the University of California, provided, at the Atoms for Peace Conference at Geneva, what might have been a chemical engineer's diagram showing every stage of the living plant's mechanism for converting carbon dioxide from the air into sucrose, and the carbohydrates of our diet. The Russian, Dr. A. M. Kuzin, reported on work extending the process of photosynthesis to the proteins and amino acids. They had also begun to decipher chlorophyll itself.

Here we have glimpses of The Grand Design—from the heart of the sun to the heart of the cell.

10. THE LIFE SECRET

Atomic research holds even more sensational possibilities than man-created food—the secret of life itself. Only it is not the study of atomic energy in this case but the study of the arrangement of atoms in the molecules of chemical compounds—the province of the crystallographer. The center of interest is DNA (deoxyribonucleic acid) one of the basic chemicals of the living cells. The biochemists, the physicists and geneticists (because DNA is a key to heredity and why you are you) are working together. They know the structure of this vital molecule—it is like a coiled spring—and they know the position of the respective atoms, and they think they know how, by attracting elemental atoms, the chemical reproduces itself. And reproduction, whether of an organism or a chemical, is what a natural scientist would interpret as life.

A long way short of producing test-tube babies from laboratory chemicals, this line of investigation may help to explain the mechanism of heredity and, much more important for suffering humanity, shed a light on the sinister secrets of cancer.

Part Nine

VICTORY OVER PAIN

> And the Lord God caused a deep sleep
> to fall upon Adam, and he slept: and he
> took one of his ribs, and closed up the
> flesh instead thereof.
>
> —GENESIS ii: 21.

1. "BIG CHIEF LAUGHING GAS"

The name of Sam Colt is usually associated with permanent unconsciousness but before he patented the revolver
he *nearly* discovered anesthetics.

It happened in this way. Samuel Colt was part owner
of a Penny Museum in Cincinnati, in the 1830s. He had
conceived the idea of a revolver but did not have the
money to complete the patents. As a youth he had traveled
the countryside with a side show which he set up in the
public squares or the fair grounds and in which he demonstrated the effects of nitrous oxide—the "laughing gas"
the strange properties of which Sir Humphry Davy had
discovered thirty years before (April 17, 1799). His per-
formance included using the laughing gas on himself and
then inviting the spectators to join in—for their own
"laughing gas" amusement and for the amusement of the
onlookers.

When he was in need of the money for the patents he
thought again of laughing gas as a quick money-maker.
This time he decided to stage a more elaborate show.
He hired six Red Indians and advertised the fact that he
was going to put them under the 'fluence. The hall was
crowded with men and their lady friends—the men armed
to protect the women against the reversion to type of the
"savage" redskins. Colt, because he had not had a dress
rehearsal, was equally apprehensive when he administered
the laughing gas. He gave the appropriate dose, which
had always worked in the past, to each of the six redskins and waited for their whoops and their exhilarated

war dance. Instead, they all became unconscious. The audience had not paid their admission to see a group of sleeping Indians. Colt, the master showman, quickly administered the gas in the same proportions to a blacksmith, who reacted as was expected and chased Sam around the stage. In the commotion they toppled the seated Indians like ninepins and the "savages" woke up dazedly. The audience was quite appreciative—they thought it was all part of the act—but Colt was mystified. He decided that laughing gas was an unreliable form of entertainment and abandoned it.

What he failed to recognize in the condition of the Indians was that he had produced complete anesthesia—painless sleep. As bitter, and bloody, experience had already shown in the case of "firewater," Red Indians react to much smaller doses of certain drugs than Anglo-Saxon blacksmiths.

Although Colt missed his place in medical history, another traveling showman, Gardner Quincy Colton, did not. After a brief study of medicine in which he learned the properties of, once again, nitrous oxide, Colton became a self-appointed "professor," traveling the country and demonstrating chemical marvels. He could attract great audiences and his "box office" often amounted to over $500 a performance.

On December 10, 1844, Colton gave an exhibition of laughing gas in the city of Hartford, Connecticut. After he had explained the effects of the gas he invited some of the audience to come onto the stage and inhale it. Among those who came forward was Dr. Horace Wells, a local dentist, and also a young man by the name of Cooley.

Cooley inhaled the gas, and while under its influence careered around the stage and banged his legs against some wooden settees. As he sat down next to Dr. Wells the latter said to him: "You must have hurt yourself." "No," said Cooley and then began to feel some pain and discovered that his legs were lacerated and covered with blood. He said that he had felt no pain until the effects of the gas wore off.

According to Colton's account, Dr. Wells came up to him afterwards and said, "Why cannot a man have a tooth extracted under gas and not feel it?" Colton replied that he did not know.

2. "HUMBUG"

Early next morning (December 1, 1844) Wells called to collect Colton. The "professor" brought along a supply of the gas in a rubber bag fitted with a tube and a wooden spigot. In Wells's dental surgery they joined Wells's associate Riggs, as well as the Cooley who had damaged his legs the night before.

The dentist sat in his own operating chair. He took in his mouth the rubber tube which Colton handed him and the spigot was turned. Riggs waited until the showman had given somewhat more gas than he usually administered in producing the exhilarating effects in his demonstrations, and until Wells was apparently unconscious. Riggs proceeded to extract a molar from the dentist's jaw. When Wells regained consciousness and was shown the tooth he exclaimed "It is the greatest discovery ever made; I did not feel so much as the prick of a pin!"

Wells immediately obtained Colton's agreement to show him all that he knew about the preparation of the gas and discovered the laboratory apparatus which would be needed.

Within a month Wells went to Boston to see his former partner, William T. G. Morton. Together Morton and Wells went to consult Charles T. Jackson, who was a well-known chemist and geologist. While Morton was prepared to believe Wells's experience Jackson pooh-poohed it. But Morton had connections at the Massachusetts General Hospital and he persuaded John Collins Warren, the most eminent surgeon of his day, to allow Wells to give a demonstration. Warren, whose name was later to bulk so large in the story of anesthetics, obviously did not believe in the claims of Wells. He introduced him to the class who were waiting to see the demonstration by saying: "There is a gentleman here who *pretends* that he has got something which will destroy pain in a surgical operation. He wants to address you. If any of you would like to hear him, you can do so."

Wells made a few halting remarks to his intimidating audience and then asked for a volunteer on whom to demonstrate. He gave the gas to his patient, took his forceps and proceeded to pull out the tooth. For some reason—perhaps because, in his nervousness, he had not waited long enough for the gas to take effect, or had not given sufficient of it—the volunteer yelled. The students in the audience jeered, hissed and shouted "Humbug!" Wells was shouldered out of the operating theater.

Wells realized that he had bungled the operation but did not lose faith in the gas itself. He continued successfully to practice painless dentistry and acquired a large clientele. Some forty citizens of Hartford later gave sworn testimonies that during 1845 Wells had extracted their teeth without pain.

3. "ETHER, AND EXCISING TUMOR: $2"

Before we return to two other characters whom we have already met, Morton and Jackson, let us make a journey to Jefferson, Georgia, to meet the town physician. It is around Christmas time 1841.

In the office of the doctor, Crawford Williamson Long, are four students. Long was only twenty-seven years of age and the students were between nineteen and twenty-one. They were discussing the effects of nitrous oxide, which was then not only the amusement of the traveling showman but also the party game of the Bright Young People. They were badgering the doctor to make them some of the gas. What happened is best described in the words of Crawford Long himself.

"I informed them that I had no apparatus for preparing or preserving the gas, but that I had a medicine (sulfuric ether) which would produce equally exhilarating effects; that I had inhaled myself, and considered it as safe as the nitrous oxide. One of the company stated, that he had inhaled ether while at school, and was willing to inhale it now. The company were all anxious to witness its effects. I gave it first to the gentleman who had previously inhaled it, then inhaled it myself, and afterwards gave it to all persons present. They were so much pleased with the exhilarating effects of the ether, that they afterwards inhaled it frequently, and induced others to do so, and its inhalation soon became quite fashionable in this county, and in fact extended from this place through several counties in this part of Georgia."

Long himself found that when he emerged from ether intoxication, as he called it, he would find that his arms

and hands were severely bruised or wounded. But he had
been quite unconscious of feeling any pain at the time of
the accidents. He saw that his friends while under the
effects would often fall with a thud which would have, or
should have, hurt them badly.

Among Long's patients was a young man named James
M. Venable, who had two tumors on the back of his neck.
Venable had himself been among those who had enjoyed
the amusement of inhaling ether and Long suggested to
him, from his own experience, that perhaps under its influence an operation could be carried out without pain.
The patient agreed to try the experiment and to have
one of the tumors removed.

The ether was given to him on a towel and, when he
was under the influence, Long cut out the tumor. It was
about half an inch in diameter.

Venable continued to inhale the ether during the operation and was surprised when he was shown the tumor.
He had not felt the slightest pain during the operation.

That, the first operation under gaseous anesthetic, appears in Long's ledger as the entry: "James Venable,
1842, ether and excising tumor, $2."

In the bitter controversies which followed in later years,
and which reached the floor of Congress itself, the fact
that Long carried out the first operation could not be
rebutted. But the fact remains that because he himself
did not publicize his discovery of the effects of ether and
its use, Long must take a diminished place in the history
of anesthesia—diminished, because a discovery of this
kind is only valid when it acquires general application.
Long's explanation of his reticence did him credit. He
said in testimony in later years that he was anxious before making any publication to try ether in a sufficient
number of cases fully to satisfy himself that the effect was
produced by the ether and was not induced by the imagination or by any special resistance to pain in the patient.

4. "MONOMANIAC"

That was scientifically proper and professionally modest
but if he had been more forthcoming in 1842 he might
have helped to avoid the disgraceful and indeed tragic
controversies which arose over the priorities of the discovery.

The controversies involved three people—Wells, Morton and Jackson. Wells, convinced of the values of nitrous oxide, had turned to his friend Morton and together they had seen Jackson.

Charles Thomas Jackson, born at Plymouth, Massachusetts, in 1805, emerges from history as a monomaniac. That in fact was the term applied to him by Samuel F. B. Morse, the inventor of the electric telegraph, when Jackson claimed that invention for himself. He also claimed to have discovered guncotton after it had been announced by C. F. Schönbein. And he tried to "muscle in" on the credit due to Beaumont for his researches into the workings of the stomach.

This attempt at piracy is itself an extraordinary incident. Beaumont was touring with St. Martin, the Canadian who had a "window in his stomach," exhibiting him before various medical societies. He had left some gastric fluid in Boston with Jackson, who was a very able chemist and who had been asked to analyze the properties of the fluid. Beaumont was under orders to proceed as an army surgeon to the West and was taking St. Martin with him. Jackson proceeded to petition the Secretary of War insisting that Dr. Beaumont should be compulsorily stationed at Boston until Jackson could complete his investigations. The circular was signed by over 200 members of Congress. Jackson had never consulted Beaumont as to his wishes and it is quite clear, from his subsequent behavior, that, if the request had been granted, which it was not, Jackson would certainly have claimed for himself Beaumont's physiological discoveries.

That was what had happened in the case of Morse. Morse and Jackson were fellow passengers on a voyage from France, of forty days and nights, in 1832.

Jackson had bought an electromagnet, along with other electrical equipment, in Paris, and he entertained the passengers with demonstrations of electricity. Morse remarked to Jackson on the voyage: "If the presence of electricity can be made visible in any part of the circuit, I see no reason why intelligence may not be transmitted instantaneously by electricity." Forthwith Morse started to make sketches of the invention which was to be so momentous and which he patented in 1837. Jackson in later years claimed that he had been responsible for the discovery, but Morse had been familiar with the electro-

magnet since 1824 and all that had happened on the
voyage had been that his imagination had been stimulated.

Jackson's intervention in the history of anesthesia is a
similar piece of poaching. As has been mentioned, he
derided Wells's idea of using nitrous oxide for surgical
operations. But Morton, inspired by Wells's experience,
was anxious to pursue the use of gas in his dental practice. It is true that Jackson suggested to Morton that he
should use ether in extracting a tooth. It is, however,
manifestly untrue that Morton was merely acting as Jackson's agent.

5. "YOUR PATIENT IS READY"

On the evening of September 30, 1846, a patient with an
ulcerated tooth called on Morton at his Boston dental office. He was in great agony but was afraid of the pain of
the extraction. He asked Morton whether he could not
mesmerize him.

This was the opportunity Morton had been looking for.
He told the patient, Eben H. Frost, that he had "something better than mesmerism." He took some ether and
called on his assistant Dr. Hayden to bring a lamp. He
poured the fluid ether onto a folded handkerchief and
gave it to Frost to hold beneath his nose. The patient
inhaled and in less than a minute his hand dropped into
his lap. Morton swiftly extracted the tooth while Hayden
held the lamp close to the mouth. This was a perilous
thing to do because the ether fumes might have ignited.
The patient did not as much as stir.

When Frost revived, the dentist, fully aware of the
possibilities, and with an eye to history, promptly got
him to sign a certificate in which he testified that he had
had the tooth painlessly removed. This was countersigned
by witnesses. The next day there appeared a notice in the
Boston Daily Journal which stated:

"Last evening, as we were informed by a gentleman
who witnessed the operation, an ulcerated tooth was extracted from the mouth of an individual, without giving
the slightest pain. He was put into a kind of sleep, by
inhaling a preparation, the effects of which lasted for
about three-quarters of a minute, just long enough to extract the tooth."

Morton took the businesslike precaution of not disclosing what the "preparation" was.

Within a week Morton was offering his method and his "preparation" for trial at Massachusetts General Hospital. This was a bold thing to do because he went again to Warren, the surgeon, to whom he had introduced Wells and who had witnessed the fiasco of the demonstration of nitrous oxide. Somehow, however, he persuaded Warren to give him an opportunity of administering gas for an operation.

The scene which follows belongs to the great drama of medicine: the patient, Gilbert Abbott, with a tumor on his jaw, was in the surgical pit of the hospital operating theater, which was jammed to the ceiling with students and doctors. The great surgeon Warren was there to operate, but the principal character, Morton, had not arrived when the curtain had been up for fifteen minutes. With professorial humor, Warren turned to the assembly and said, "I presume he is otherwise engaged," and in the dutiful roar of laughter which followed Morton arrived. He made his bow and with Warren's permission withdrew to prepare his apparatus. He was still intent on keeping his "preparation" secret and had masked the recognizable smell of ether with perfumes. He saturated a sponge with the liquid and inserted it into a glass globe which he corked and brought with him to the theater.

"Well, sir!" said Warren sarcastically, "your patient is ready."

Morton put the tube to the patient's lips and told him to breathe in and out of the globe through his mouth. Abbott obeyed. At first his face flushed and his arms and legs jerked but Morton kept the globe steady and the tube in Abbott's mouth until, after three or four minutes, the gas took effect.

"Sir," said Morton bowing to Warren, *"your* patient is ready."

The surgeon wielded his knife and the gathering braced itself for the usual screams of anguish from a patient exposed to the surgical tortures of the times.

No sound issued from Abbott. Quickly Warren completed his operation. The wound was closed, the patient's face was washed and gradually he emerged from the effects. He was questioned. He said he had felt no pain but thought of something blunt scratching his cheek.

Turning to the assembly the surgeon said: "Gentlemen, *this* is no humbug."

6. *"YANKEE DODGE"*

Two months later, at University College Hospital in London, ether was to have its European premiere. Again the setting is a crowded amphitheater with the great Robert Liston prepared to operate. The anesthetist was William Squire, the son of the chemist who had prepared the ether. In that audience was Joseph Lister, whose "safe surgery" (through antiseptics) was presently to be added to "painless surgery" (through anesthetics). Like Warren, Liston approached the experiment with typical professorial skepticism.

He turned to the gallery and said: "We are going to try a Yankee dodge today, gentlemen, for making men insensible."

Liston in his time was a living legend. A giant of a man, his strength was prodigious. In amputating a thigh, he would use the grip of his left hand as a tourniquet to compress the artery, while he wielded the scalpel or the saw with his right. If he needed a spare hand he would hold the saw in his teeth. He worked so fast that students were warned not to sneeze or they would miss the operation. His nerves were of tempered steel but even they twanged like fiddle strings under the stresses of the agonies of the suffering patients, strapped to the operating table. If only the Yankee dodge would work . . .

The patient, Frederick Churchill, a butler, was having his thigh amputated through the fault of Liston himself, although the surgeon would not reproach himself. Churchill had fallen and injured his tibia and a discharging sinus had formed. He was sent to London's greatest surgeon, who probed the sinus, made the incision, put his uncouth finger into the wound, felt the bone and plugged it up. The result—blood poisoning. The only answer—amputation.

So there was the unfortunate Churchill, sweating with apprehension, while the stage was set. At length Squire (presently to be known as what O. W. Holmes first called an "anesthetist") said: "He is ready now, sir."

Sir R. Reynolds, who was present, wrote: "I took out my watch to count the time. Liston's knife flashed in the air, and the leg was on the floor in six and twenty seconds. Liston turned to his students and said, 'This Yankee dodge, gentlemen, beats mesmerism."

7. *"SO PRECIOUS A GIFT . . ."*

That was December twenty-first. Within thirteen days— on January 2, 1847—the medical journal *The Lancet* carried a sinister letter:

"I take this earliest opportunity of giving notice, through the medium of your columns, to the medical profession, and to the public at large, that the process of procuring insensibility to pain by the administration of the vapor ether to the lungs, employed by Mr. Liston, is patented for England and the colonies, and that no person can use that process, or a similar one, without infringing upon rights legally secured to others."

It was signed by James A. Dorr, Morton's agent in London. The letter included a justification of this attempt to exploit what Warren had described as "so precious a gift. . . . Unrestrained and free as God's own sunshine, it has gone forth to cheer and gladden the earth. . . ."

"I cannot see why the individual who, by industry and skill, invents or discovers the means of diminishing, or, as in this instance, annihilating human suffering, is not full as much entitled to compensation as he who makes an improvement in the manufacture of woollen or other fabrics. Indeed he is entitled to greater compensation— he has conferred upon mankind a greater benefit. . . ."

That was Morton's line and he was sticking to it. Within a fortnight of the epoch-making episode at Massachusetts General Hospital, he and Jackson sought a patent for *Letheon,* but all the perfumes of Arabia could not deceive the medical profession, which recognized it as sulfuric ether, then used in practice for catarrh and whooping cough.

Some idea of what Morton hoped to make out of it can be gathered from the fact that he licensed Dr. Fisk of Salem to have the exclusive use in Essex County, Massachusetts, for $850 for five years. On the same basis for the whole of the United States, with a population of twenty-three millions, Morton's share of the U.S. patent royalties would have been $356,000—apart from world rights.

Jackson, whose greed for money was less than his greed for glory, quickly renounced his half-share and settled for ten per cent of the patent royalties, which never materialized because the patent claim was untenable. Instead, he wrote to Elie de Beaumont in Paris and persuaded him to present his claims to be the exclusive discoverer of anesthesia before the French Academy. He never mentioned Morton. He also delivered a paper before the American Academy of Arts and Sciences, and post-hasted this to Paris, conveying the impression to the whole of Europe that the American Academy had endorsed his claim.

When the Paris Medical Institute awarded a prize of 2,500 francs to Jackson and a similar amount to Morton, the latter refused to accept it, insisting on the full credit.

8. "AN UNSPEAKABLE EVIL"

Meanwhile, Horace Wells was champing at the acclaim which had greeted his old partner, Morton. His wife later declared that his discovery had been to his family "an unspeakable evil"; it wrecked a happy home; it ruined a successful practice (because of his obsession) and finally cost her husband his life.

Early in 1847, Wells, still only thirty-two years of age, sailed for Paris to counter the claims of the other two. He received a sympathetic hearing and he was feted as a great hero. His account of his priority was submitted by an American dentist in Paris, C. Starr Brewster, to the Paris Medical Society, which repented its precipitate recognition of Jackson and Morton. But before its findings were made public the impatient Wells had returned to New York. His self-experiments with gas had undermined his constitution. He "topped them off" with trials of chloroform and hastened the final tragedy.

In a letter dated January 12, 1848, Brewster wrote from Paris informing him that the Paris Medical Society had voted him the honor of the first discoverer of "the use of vapors or gases whereby surgical operations could be performed without pain . . . and to the last day of time suffering humanity must bless the name of Horace Wells."

Before it reached Wells, he was dead. He was caught in the act of hurling vitriol at some New York street-walkers, was arrested and sent to the Tombs prison to await sentence. Overwhelmed by shame he wrote a letter to his wife asking forgiveness for what he was about to do; took the remains of the chloroform from the orgy which had affected his mind; and, as the chloroform dulled his senses, his last conscious act was to slash the femoral artery in his thigh.

In July 1868, a furiously embittered Morton returned from Washington from his perennial fight for a Congressional appropriation of $100,000 in personal recognition of his discovery. He was in the throes of a nervous break-down. Two doctors were called. They pronounced his condition serious; installed a trained nurse; ordered blood-letting, ice packs and absolute rest.

The moment they left, Morton jumped into his buggy and drove wildly up Broadway and into Central Park. At the upper end of the park, he jumped out, ran to the lake and pushed his head into the water. He was hauled out and persuaded to get back into his buggy. But he had driven only a short distance when he leaped down again, jumped over a fence and collapsed unconscious. A few hours later he was dead.

Jackson, still trying desperately to climb on the band-wagon, had made public another "discovery"—the use of ether as what we would now call a "tranquilizer" in the treatment of obstreperous mental cases. He reported its successful use in cases treated in McLean Asylum.

McLean Asylum was where he himself spent the last seven years of his life—as a patient, and there is no record that ether did him any good.

Crawford Long, who had been so discreet about his surgical success with ether four and a half years before Morton's demonstration with the same gas, became embroiled in the controversy. His main contribution was his evidence, which, submitted to Congress through Senator Dawson, prevented an award being made to Morton.

He had not prospered either. The Civil War had beggared his Georgian patients and he had a large but unremunerative practice.

In 1877, he was attending a woman in difficult labor. He administered ether, and delivered the child. As he handed the baby to the nurse, he collapsed and died of an apoplectic stroke.

9. "I AM AN ANGEL"

Now let us adjourn to Scotland. A young professor of midwifery at the University of Edinburgh was attending an unusual party. His name was James Y. Simpson, a village baker's son, who at the age of twenty-eight had been appointed to the professorship which, on this date (November 4, 1847), he had held for eight years. One of his professorial colleagues, Dr. Miller, was present and left an account:

"On returning home after a weary day's work, Dr. Simpson with his two friends and assistants, Drs. Keith and Duncan, sat down to a hazardous work in Dr. Simpson's dining-room. Having inhaled several substances, but without much effect, it occurred to Dr. Simpson to try some ponderous material which he had formerly set aside on a lumber table, and which, on account of its great weight, he had hitherto regarded as of no likelihood whatever. *That* happened to be a small bottle of chloroform. It was searched for and found under a heap of wastepaper. And with each tumbler newly charged, the inhalers resumed their vocation. Immediately, an unwonted hilarity seized the party: they became bright-eyed, very happy, and very locquacious. The conversation was of unusual intelligence and quite charmed the listeners—who included some ladies of the family and a naval officer.

"But suddenly there was a talk of sounds being heard, like the clatter of a cotton mill, louder and louder; a moment more then all was quiet—and then CRASH! The inhaling party slipped off their chairs and flopped on to the floor unconscious."

After that, the rest of the party insisted on joining in. Miss Petrie, a niece of Dr. Simpson's, wishing to prove that she could be as brave as any man, inhaled the chloroform, folded her arms on her breast and "went under" exclaiming "I'm an angel! Oh, I'm an angel!"

Simpson never competed for the credit of discovering *anesthesia*. He was content to have discovered the values of *chloroform* and to have employed them in the relief of the pains of childbirth. He acquired honors—including a baronetcy, for which he chose as his coat-of-arms the Aesculapian serpent and the motto Victo dolore (Victory over Pain).

His battle was not with rivals but with bigots. The clergy thundered from their pulpits against his use of chloroform in childbirth—"In sorrow thou shalt bring forth children" (Gen. iii:16). And one of his fiercest battles was with Dr. Meigs of Philadelphia, who, having previously invoked the great name of Simpson in his controversy with Oliver Wendell Holmes over clean hands in midwifery, now assailed his painless childbirth. "Pain of childbirth," said Meigs, "is a desirable, salutary, and conservative manifestation of the life-force."

Simpson was a redoubtable debater. He pointed out to Meigs that nature had not provided railways and suggested that the next time Meigs traveled to New York or Baltimore, he ought to walk. He also prophesied that one day the canal would be built across the Isthmus of Panama but that there would be opposition because God had put mountains and rocks between the two seas.

With the clergy in his own country, he joined polemical battle, rebutting their arguments on their own theological ground, going back to the Greek and the Hebrew, and arguing that "sorrow" was not "pain" but "labour," and resoundingly demolishing their case by invoking Genesis ii:21: "And the Lord God caused a deep sleep to fall upon Adam, and he slept; and He took one of his ribs, and closed up the flesh instead thereof." God was the first anesthetist.

In February 1957, 110 years later, over radio which spanned the globe and on television sets, the world heard the papal sanction and justification of the use, and limits of use, of anesthetics.

10. "BY ROYAL APPOINTMENT"

Simpson won his battle, not by his eloquence entirely but because Queen Victoria decided to have her son Prince Leopold with the help of chloroform.

The anesthetic, "by Royal Appointment," was administered to the Queen, not by Simpson but by Dr. John Snow, who has a very special place in medical history, not just because he assisted at a royal lying-in but because, as well as developing the techniques of surgical anesthesia, he played a momentous part in the history of public health.

Coming out of hospital one day, Snow met a druggist whom he patronized and wished him "Good morning!"

"Don't detain me, doctor," cried the druggist. "I am giving ether, here, there and everywhere, and am getting quite into an ether practice."

This gave Snow cause to think. In 1841, when he was twenty-eight, he had written on artificial respiration for newborn children and had devised an apparatus. He was familiar, therefore, with "pneumatics"—medical treatment with gases. After his encounter with the druggist he studied the behavior of ether and devised safe methods for its administration. When he was summoned to the palace he was Britain's leading anesthetist, who had worked out scientifically the application of gases. He made scientific measurements of dosages and calculated the weight and amount of blood in a patient, and the physiological reactions, to the point where he could measure precisely the amount of anesthetic which would produce insensibility for a given time. (He could have told Samuel Colt why his Red Indians became unconscious with the same amount of nitrous oxide which made the blacksmith "hopping mad.")

John Snow, and the Broad Street Pump, have a conspicuous place in the development of modern sanitation and preventive medicine.

The Public Health Service, it has been said, should regard cholera as its greatest benefactor. Long before Koch had discovered the *vibrio,* the micro-organism responsible, the onset of cholera in prosperous communities had made the High-and-the-Mighty aware that this was a risk which they shared with the Low-and-the-Humble, and that somehow the whole community must be protected, since, in this respect at least, riches could not buy privileged immunity.

In 1854 cholera was amuck in London. The officials were in despair. There was one plague spot where, within a radius of 250 yards, 500 victims had died within ten days. Panic was setting in and it looked as though Londoners were to flee the city as in the days of medieval plagues.

While the vestrymen of the parish of St. James's were in session, a doctor insisted on an interview. It was John Snow, and he had one suggestion to make—that they *take off the handle of the pump* in Broad Street. This sounded ridiculous at a time when even the chief medical officer of England still believed that infectious diseases were spread by effluvia and miasmata. But the situation was so desperate that the vestrymen agreed; the handle was removed and the cholera plague disappeared.

Snow, who had encountered cholera as a young medical assistant near Newcastle-on-Tyne, had retained his interest even when he became a successful and fashionable London anesthetist. He had visited the plague spot in St. James's and had found that a cartridge factory, which drew tubs of drinking water from the pump, was ravaged by the disease but that the workmen at the local brewery, who drank malted liquor instead of water, were not affected. The householders in the vicinity, using the pump water, had cholera; the paupers in the local almshouse, which drew its water from its own well, had none. And so, by process of elimination, he decided that the pump was delivering cholera-infested water; and it was so. In that incident doctors made the discovery that cholera was a water-borne disease and that water purification was necessary.

11. *"A LITTLE EAU DE COLOGNE"*

So far we have been discussing generalized anesthesia, but it is not necessary in many cases to produce complete insensibility when a local painkiller can be used.

One night Benjamin Ward Richardson, a successful British physician, went to a ball with his wife. He had been working all day in his laboratory trying to find some way of isolating pain:

"A young lady with whom I was about to dance let a little eau-de-Cologne fall on my forehead, by blowing it briskly through a small tube. The cold produced was intense and pinching the bit of skin affected by it I found that it was benumbed. 'Thank you!' I said, and seized upon the fact."

Next day he went to his laboratory and studied the effects on the skin of the rapid evaporation of volatile liquids. He then produced local insensibility by freezing the part with an ether spray. This spray, from that date (1867) was the only known method of local anesthesia until the coming of cocaine in 1884.

12. *"MAMA COCA"*

The worshipful title held by the queens of the Incas was "Mama Coca." The qualities of the coca plant were prized by the Incas as a solace second only to women.

Tales of prodigies of endurance are told of the Peruvian Indians, who, while holding a few leaves of coca mixed with ashes in their mouths, can run up mountains and forgo food and sleep.

The properties of this Divine Plant of the Incas were examined by Albert Niemann, an assistant of the great German chemist Wöhler at Gottingen. In 1860 he crystallized the active principle and called it *cocaine*. Although others found that hypodermic injections of cocaine could rob the injected part of all sensation, the medical profession neglected it for fully a quarter of a century.

13. *FREUDIAN SLIP*

Then cocaine came to the profession's notice through a circumstance involving one who was to become famous in an entirely different branch of medicine—Sigmund Freud.

A young colleague of Freud's in Vienna had become an opium addict through trying to relieve the pain in an amputated thumb. He wanted to free himself from the addiction and he consulted Freud, who tried to fight the addiction by substituting cocaine. Anxious to know more about the physiological effects of the drug, Freud invited another colleague, Carl Koller, to join him in experiments.

It is one of the freaks of medical history that Freud, not Koller, might have discovered cocaine as a local anesthetic if sex had not reared its head. Freud collected the few grams of the crystalline cocaine which then existed in the world but, in the middle of the experiments, Freud had an urge to visit his fiancée, whom he had not seen for two years. When he returned from his holiday, he found that Koller had made decisive experiments on an animal's eye, and had demonstrated them at an ophthalmological congress in Heidelberg. There, a patient suffering from glaucoma had had a few drops of cocaine given in the eye. A surgeon then inserted a probe into the cornea. The patient, fully conscious, felt no pain.

The advances in local anesthesia were made largely in America (Koller emigrated there) and, in particular, by William Stewart Halsted, of Johns Hopkins University, who demonstrated (1885) that anesthesia of almost any part of the body could be induced by drug injection. In the same year, James Leonard Corning, a New York surgeon, introduced spinal anesthesia (injections of cocaine into the spinal cord), and G. W. Crile of Chile, Ohio, combined spinal anesthesia with general anesthesia, thereby reducing the shock of operation—a technique which Harvey Cushing, one of the greatest of all nerve surgeons, was to perfect and employ in his outstanding work.

Today, the practice of anesthesia is a science in itself. From the slap-happy use of laughing gas to the refinements of general anesthetics today, from the cocaine-in-the-eye to the use of *curare* (like cocaine, a South American drug) to relax the tensed muscles of modern man (tensed even when he is asleep) there has been a procession of pain-quelling drugs. The changes can be rung to suit each case. The patient is studied by the anesthetist for his possible reactions as thoroughly as his symptoms are studied by the surgeon who is to operate.

Thanks to a strolling showman (as Oliver Wendell Holmes might have said, when he realized the role of "Professor" Gardner Quincy Colton) the present-day surgeon can enter parts of the body where Liston, however fast his knife, could never have dreamed of entering—into the recesses of the brain, the chest cavity, the heart, the lungs and the great blood vessels.

14. PANTHEON OF IMMORTALS

More than a painless and submissive patient, more than aseptic operating theaters, bereft of germs, and more than deft fingers and subtle anatomical knowledge have been needed to make possible modern surgical miracles and the reprieves from a death which would have been certain only a few brief years ago.

There are other galleries in the Pantheon of the Immortals into which we must glance in passing. Let us see them as episodes like a series of dioramas.

(A) Roentgen

The setting is the dining room of an inconspicuous professor of physics at the University of Würzburg, Bavaria. The year is 1895. Frau Roentgen is cross, as any long-suffering wife would be—her Wilhelm has been thoroughly annoying. For the past few days he has been more than usually absent-minded; normally, he does not speak much but at least he should answer when he is spoken to; his poet's beard has been uncombed and untidy. To-night's behavior is the last straw. All afternoon, Frau Roentgen has been slaving over a hot stove conjuring up his favorite meal and now he has eaten it, without comment and without relish; it might just have been bread and cheese. His wife is angry and all the angrier because he does not even notice that she is angry. So she loses her temper and really scolds him. Wilhelm is not an inconsiderate husband and, contritely, he explains that he really has something on his mind—something which is difficult to explain and something difficult to believe. Maybe she would like to see it for herself. . . .

And so Frau Roentgen was the first person, apart from her husband, to see the phenomenon of X rays. One doubts very much whether she thought, then, that it was sufficient excuse for a wasted supper. All she saw was a dim glow in the pitch-darkness of the laboratory, but to Wilhelm it had a profound meaning.

He had been studying the effect on fluorescent salts of the radiations from a Crookes tube. Sir William Crookes had made a vacuum tube shaped like an airship; towards the bulbous end he had set a metal cross. When an electric current was applied to the electrode at the mouth of the tube a beam of "something" passed to the cross, which was his other electrode. The "something" made the glass at the bulbous end glow and cast a clear-cut shadow of the metal cross. Roentgen was pursuing the "something," and was using barium-platino-cyanide crystals to see if "it" provoked fluorescence. "It" did, but, to test his experiment, he enclosed the tube in a container of blackened cardboard which would prevent the tube from emitting any light. Yet it still caused the salts to glow—even at a distance of twelve feet. It was "agin natur'." There must be an invisible "light" coming from the dark lantern.

Years later, he was asked by Sir James Mackenzie, the famous heart specialist, what he thought when he noticed this.

"Think?" said Roentgen, in the spirit of the true scientist, "I did not think! I investigated."

He put a dense object on top of a sealed wooden box on top of a sealed wooden box in which he enclosed a photographic plate and he got an image of the object on the plate. Similarly, he could photograph the skeleton of his own hand. If the pressure in the tube was low, he could get the bones with only a faint shadow of the flesh.

Roentgen was a physicist but his first paper was read to the Medical Society of Würzburg—because he had seen its surgical significance, as a practical aid to surgeons. He called them X rays.

(B) Marie Curie

In September 1897, Marie Curie, formerly Marie Sklodovski of Warsaw, has just given birth to a daughter, Irene. And, as she keeps house in Paris and bathes the baby, scrubs the pans and worries how her husband's poor stipend as chief of the laboratory at the School of Physics and Chemistry can meet the housekeeping bills for three, she wonders whether she will ever be able to get her degree as a doctor of science. She debates her subject for her thesis in her mind.

Henri Becquerel, professor of physics, had done something rather like Roentgen—only the other way round. He had wondered whether fluorescent salts themselves might not give off such rays. He had prepared salts of uranium and had wrapped the element in black paper, placed it on silver foil and put the lot on a photographic plate. Sure enough! There was the blotch of the uranium image. He had discovered spontaneous radioactivity.

Marie Curie, looking for her thesis subject, jumps to a conclusion—against all the tenets that the atom is the ultimate, indivisible, particle of matter—and decides that the Becquerel Effect is some explosive property of the atom.

But that would not be significant if such radiation was merely an eccentric and rather feeble characteristic of uranium. So Marie Curie, nursing her infant Irene, makes a decision (momentous for mankind): she will examine *every known element*.

Her only laboratory is the glassed-in storeroom adjoining her husband's laboratory. Presently she finds another element with the ray-emitting characteristics of uranium —thorium. Then, in addition to the study of the simple elements, she turns to the minerals in which they are encountered in nature and she finds certain chunks—notably pitchblende from Bohemia—which give evidence of more intense activity. But, *mon dieu!* has she not examined every known element? If there is one that behaves differently it must be a new element. But, *ma chérie* (protest the savants, in avuncular condescension), that is a foolishness. Perhaps, but she will put her preliminary findings on record just the same, and, jeopardizing her doctorate, she pronounces to the Academy—just the possibility, no more.

Truly, it is heartbreaking—so elusive. And backbreaking, for, to reduce her samples, she must stand over a great caldron, stirring the pitchblende, like a washerwoman stirring clothes. And just when it seems already found, it sneaks away, plays a trick. Can it be? Yes, it is! Not one new element, but two! And here is the first Polonium, which she names for her native Poland, from which as a rebel against the tsar she is a refugee. But there is more "kick" in that other still to be found.

Marie keeps a journal. On one page she writes: "I took eight pounds of fruit and the same weight of crystallized sugar, boiled for ten minutes, passed the mixture through a fine sieve and obtained fourteen pots of very good jelly —not transparent but it set perfectly."

Later we find her writing: "Irene can walk very well and no longer goes on all fours." The date is October 17, 1898.

On January 6, 1899, she makes a proud entry: "Irene has 15 teeth."

And, in the interval, there is another entry: "We believe that the new radioactive substance contains a new element to which we propose to give the name RADIUM."

Radium. One of the greatest discoveries of all time. The element which set Rutherford and others asking, "Why does Marie's radium give off rays?" and to find in the ultimate answer the atomic bomb and atomic industrial energy.

True, today radium is discarded with the tailings from the crushing and extraction of uranium, the atomic fuel. Radium, once worth a fabulous amount as a treatment for cancer, has now been replaced by man-made sources —radioactive cobalt, radiostrontium, and radiocesium. But, apart from Marie Curie's pioneer discovery, for which she got the Nobel Prize, those man-made healers can date their pedigree to 1933, when that selfsame Irene, whose teeth ranked in maternal importance with radium, and her husband Frédéric Joliot-Curie, produced artificial radioactivity by transmuting elements. They, too, won the Nobel Prize.

Today, research into disease and treatment of it are in process of being revolutionized by radioactive tracers, by products of nuclear energy. What X rays did as an external source, they can do from inside. Inject radioactive elements into a cavity of the body, pass a detector, like the scanner of a television picture, over the site and the result is a scintillation picture of the trouble.

But for forty years radium was the surgeon's answer to the intractable problem of cancer—not a completely satisfactory one but a medical benefaction just the same.

When the first results of radium treatment of cancer became known, radium became the world's most precious substance. The discoverers, Marie and her husband, Pierre, remained poor. They were approached commercially and had to decide whether freely to disclose, not their discovery, which was a scientific truth, but their techniques, or to patent them and become wealthy.

"It is impossible," said Marie Curie. "It would be against the scientific spirit. Physicists should always publish their results completely. If our discovery has a scientific future that is a circumstance from which we should not profit. If radium is to be used for the treatment of disease, it is impossible for us to take advantage of that."

"It is impossible," echoed Pierre Curie. "It would be contrary to the scientific spirit."

And having renounced all hope of gain, they mounted their bicycles and pedaled happily to the woods of Clamart.

(C) Carrel and Lindbergh

In 1935, Alexis Carrel is in Paris on holiday from the Rockefeller Institute of New York. He is relaxing in congenial company, a French-born visitor from America, where he had settled. The *joie d'esprit* of the occasion disarms him. He is expansive. After all, he is among friends, 3,000 miles away from the formalities of his post, and he has a secret he has been keeping for five years. He has, he confides, an excellent assistant. The name? Charles Lindbergh. Yes, he explains, the same Lindbergh who had flown the Atlantic.

A rash piece of gossip. The scientist has forgotten the pitcher-ears of the world press. Immediately, the telephones and cables are humming. American editors are "roasting" their Paris correspondents. Get hold of Carrel. How long has Lindbergh been working at the Rockefeller Institute? What's he up to? No good trying Carrel —he has buttoned up again. No good trying Lindbergh, refugee from the tragic notoriety of his son's kidnapping. No good trying the Rockefeller Institute—this is uncompleted research.

So the newspapers fume and speculate while the collaborators get on with their job. A strange combination— the Nobel Prize winner (1912) for his contributions to physiology and surgery, who had transplanted organs and substituted lost pieces of arteries and veins, like a plumber replacing piping, and The Lone Flyer, whose adventurous fame had obscured a real mechanical ability and a deeply serious nature.

Mechanical problems, which delighted Lindbergh, bewildered Carrel. For many years the physiologist had been wrestling with the problem of how to keep whole body organs—livers, spleens, and thyroids—alive outside the living body. He had succeeded, in laboratory mock-ups, in keeping bits of chicken heart throbbing and repairing its tissue cells. But he needed something more thorough. His dream was a machine which would show students how the pancreas actually secreted its juices and the adrenals squirted their booster chemicals into the blood.

Carrel had solved the problem up to a point. He could

feed sterile oxygen into model machines by passing it through filters to exclude bacteria, but those organisms were always sneaking through and making short shrift of the preserved organs. He needed something which would avoid this, ensure that the pumping functions of the heart were accurately reproduced, and would do what the lungs do—supply oxygen and remove the waste-products from the blood.

Lindbergh took the problem away with him to brood over it and came back with his mechanical suggestions. He cracked the basic problems and the device was constructed.

Carrel's surgical skill extracted an organ from an animal and hooked it into the glistening new apparatus. He closed the system, now germproof, and set the compressed oxygen-nitrogen-carbon-dioxide jets working to supply the motive power for the circulation system. That organ survived and so did an endless succession of others.

In his *Culture of Organs,* Alexis Carrel discussed the future possibilities of the Lindbergh pump:

"Diseased organs could be removed from the body and placed in the pump as patients are placed in hospitals. They could be treated far more energetically than within the organ, and, if cured, replanted in the patient. The thyroid extirpated in the course of an operation . . . the kidney removed for tuberculosis, or the leg amputated for osteosarcoma, would perhaps heal under the influence of an artificial medium, while living *in vitro.* The replantation would offer no difficulty as the surgical techniques for the suture of blood vessels and the transplantation of organs and limbs were developed long ago. . . ."

The day when a human uterus, with an embryo, could be thus put into a machine and produce a full-term baby has still to come, if it ever will, but Carrel's machine for physiological research has inspired surgical procedures of vital importance.

Today, machines exist which can by-pass the heart and the lungs. Artificial kidneys function outside the body. Surgical operations which would have been inconceivable a few brief years ago are now successfully carried out.

For example, the circulation of the blood through the heart is like a river going over a waterfall. To build a dam on a river, engineers would sink caissons and make detours so that the work on the site could progress. So, too, with the surgeon. To operate on the heart for any length of time, he has to have the blood redirected. This can now be done. The blood flows out of the body and back into it through a machine which keeps the blood flowing at the right pace, properly oxygenated and, if need be, reinforced by nutrient transfusions. The transparent tubes can admit ultraviolet light to keep the blood absolutely sterile, killing the germs as they pass.

With hypothermia (artificial hibernation, or cooling of the body so that its processes are slowed down) and diathermy (the electric device which makes the tissue divide and seal again at the touch of an electrode-scalpel), "impossible" operations are carried out today —"impossible" at least a few years ago because of the loss of blood, or damage of tissues through infiltration with blood, or alternatively failure of the blood supply to maintain sufficient oxygen to delicate structures like the brain.

A rather macabre comment on all this is that social clubs have been formed of people who have "died." Their hearts have stopped beating and their respiration has failed—often on the surgical operating table—and with drugs and methods now available, they have been brought back from the dead.

In case these advances give us delusions of immortality, I should quote my revered friend, the late Waldemar Kaempffert, for so long science editor of *The New York Times,* in his book *Science Today and Tomorrow:*

"The body is what the physicist calls a 'closed system,' like an automobile. Our inability to live forever lies right there. No closed system can endure unless it can inspect itself, stop corrosion, oil itself, keep itself in repair. The automobile cannot do that. But the body can—and does imperfectly. If we cannot live forever it is because of this imperfection."

We can expect much from those mechanics of the human body, the surgeons, but not too much. There is a limit to the repairs that they can do.

Part Ten

VICTORY OVER GERMS

It takes six or seven years for malaria-type mosquitoes of an area under continuous spraying to develop resistance. Consequently, if we can eradicate malaria in five years, as is possible, we may be pretty sure that we can end the spraying safely before resistance appears . . . .

—Dr. PAUL F. RUSSELL, Rockefeller Foundation, New York, in *WHO Newsletter*.

1. THE BUDDHA OF THE HUMMING MARSH

In the north of Thailand, in the district of Serapei, is the Wat Phra Norn Nong Pung. That means "The Temple of the Reclining Buddha of the Humming Swamp."

Today this is a misnomer. The Buddha still reclines, a recumbent image, sixty-five feet long and sheathed from head to foot in gold-leaf—an image so big that they had had to build the temple around it. But the swamp has ceased to hum. The mosquitoes which gave it its name no longer exist. How they disappeared is one of the most colorful stories of this age of medical miracles.

In 1949, the World Health Organization was asked by the Thai government to co-operate in a campaign of malaria control, in this region where malaria was endemic. Between 60 and 70 per cent of the population consistently suffered from the disease, which shortened their lives, robbed them of fitness, and was always liable, like a sleeping volcano of infection, to erupt into epidemics. The World Health Organization agreed to assign a team to the region, supplied with insecticides by the United Nations Children's Fund.

They appointed a Hindu malariologist, Dr. Sambasivan, as the head of the team. It was a wise choice because the difficulties were more than medical. Thailand is a devout Buddhist country. And the first of the Nine Incapabilities, the Injunctions of the Lord Buddha to his followers who would achieve Nirvana says: *He who has followed the Eightfold Path of Enlightenment is incapable of deliberately depriving a living creature of life.*

The devout Buddhist, therefore, would not choose to kill even a mosquito, although, of course, that insect does not share his scruples and is liable to kill him with malaria. Consider, then, the difficulties which confronted the doctors whose successful control of the disease depended on killing the mosquitoes. It is easy to say, "Tcha! Superstition!" But in malaria control, which depends on the co-operation of the mass of the people, their religious susceptibilities cannot be ignored; they cannot be bulldozed; they must be persuaded. That was where the Hindu upbringing of Dr. Sambasivan proved invaluable. He recognized that his work could only succeed if he could bring about an alliance between modern science and traditional religion.

He consulted the Chief Abbot of the north, an eminent Buddhist theologian, with an enlightened interest in the welfare of his people. The result was an appeal by the Chief Abbot to all Buddhists, including monks and priests, to co-operate with the doctors. The basis of the *rapprochement* was the following argument: In death there are degrees of suffering, and the sentient being, the human organism, suffers more in dying of malaria than the lesser creatures would suffer from DDT. And, although it remains a sin to kill anything, even a mosquito, the sin is qualified because its death means less suffering for men, women and children. Moreover, Buddhism is a highly personalized religion. Nobody but the individual himself can acquit or absolve him from his acts on earth, but neither is he responsible for the acts of others. And so while the truly devout could not kill a mosquito there was no personal sin in conniving at it.

With this dispensation, the international team set to work. The Buddhist monks responded by throwing open their monasteries, temples and pagodas to the doctors and their teams of DDT sprayers. The teams with their jets of liquid DDT went into the temples and sprayed the priceless mosaics and images—not because the Buddhist images had to be protected from malaria but because it was symbolic. The priests, with their shaven heads and eyebrows, swathed in their saffron togas, stood by to show their silent approval and thus to impress the villagers, whose huts had to be sprayed, with the need for similar co-operation.

Two years later, on the second anniversary of the Chief Abbot's appeal, I went into this region to see the results. The co-operation had been so complete that the monks had turned their temples into clinics, not only for malaria checks, but for the care of mothers and children. In the Temple of the Reclining Buddha of the Humming Swamp, the doctors—now Thai doctors, trained in malaria control—used an altar table as a clinical couch, and, with the Buddha smiling his golden smile upon the proceedings, they examined the children for the telltale sign of malaria—the enlarged spleen.

Among all the children whom we examined there was not one case of enlarged spleen. In the whole region there was no new case of malaria, and in all our searches of the breeding grounds we could not find a single larva of *Anopheles minimus*. In two years malaria had been banished from Serapei.

This was an occasion for a great celebration. The people of Chiengmai turned out in their thousands, and formed a great procession through the streets of the northern capital. The procession was led by the Court Dancers, exquisitely beautiful, in vivid dresses, with crowns of flowers and six-inch-long golden fingernails. With bare feet they danced through the streets, twisting to the slow rhythm and spelling out, in the "Alphabet of the Dance," legends in movements, without words. Behind them, in the miles-long procession was the "busabok," the ceremonial car, drawn by ropes. Pulling on those ropes were expectant mothers, the sick and the strong, the young and the old—pulling their way to health. And the procession moved into the great temple, where hundreds of saffron-robed monks under their scarlet parasols were assembled round their Chief Abbot. There on the lawns, in the sunlight, behind an altar smothered in flowers, was the dazzling radiant image of the Golden Buddha. The Court Dancers danced in front of the Buddha, telling, in the Alphabet of the Dance, a modern legend—the Death of the Mosquito.

This victory over the mosquito had been achieved by the modern methods of malaria control—by what is called residual spraying. The liquid insecticide, sprayed on the walls, dries off to leave a deposit which is lethal to the insect which lands on it. But a great deal more than that is involved. Much depends on the entomologist, who studies the behavior of insects.

If we take the case of Serapei, there were thirty types of mosquitoes in this region, any one of which might have been the villain. Each one had to be systematically examined. Number thirteen—*Anopheles minimus*—was found to be the carrier. In its salivary glands were found the spores of human malaria, but they had to examine every one in case the others might be carriers too. In the process, they had to train Thais in this type of research so that they, from there on, could maintain an eternal vigil, because it is always possible that a new type of carrier may appear.

Indeed, *Anopheles minimus* had originally come into Thailand with irrigation water from Burma. Although we usually associate malaria with insects that breed in stagnant waters, this one favored running water and bright sunshine, so that it bred in the canals which supplied the rice fields, and spread throughout the whole region.

Once they had identified the carrier, they then thoroughly studied all its habits. They found that the mosquito never settled higher than eight feet from the floor, that the "airstrips" from which it took off on its sorties were the walls of the huts. (Other types, in other parts, may prefer the roof thatching, for instance.) Therefore, it was necessary to spray the walls only to that height. They also found that it was mainly active between 9 o'clock at night and 5 o'clock in the morning.

The malariologists ignored the breeding places because if they killed enough adult mosquitoes they would reduce the breeding anyway. So, by wall-spraying, they disposed of the mosquito before it attacked the human, to pass on the spores of malaria to a fresh victim or to pick up the malaria from an active case.

This method, adapted to the different habits of the different types of mosquitoes, has been applied all over the world. It has been emphasized that it is *control,* not *eradication,* such as was applied in the islands of Sardinia and Cyprus. There the idea was to get rid of every mosquito and then ensure that no new mosquitoes entered the islands. But elsewhere land masses were involved, and mosquitoes do not submit to customs barriers or immigration control. The principle, therefore, was to reduce the proportion of malaria carriers so that the number of new cases would be reduced to a minimum and could be treated clinically with modern drugs. If the mosquitoes cannot pick up the malaria from human cases, they cannot pass it on, and so the disease will diminish and disappear.

That was the theory, but doctors have always been aware that the practice was fraught with danger. Once a region has been rid of malaria, a fresh outbreak, in epidemic proportions, would tear through the district like a forest fire. This could happen if a new mosquito carrier appeared, from some other quarter, and its habits were different from those against which the DDT precautions had prevailed. More serious is the appearance of resistant types of mosquitoes. Insects develop an immunity to insect poisons. It is possible to "ring the changes" by using different types of insecticide, but gradually a mosquito may be bred which will defy the lot.

This resistance is not an acquired habit—such as occurs when people eat small amounts of arsenic and become inured to the poison. This is selective breeding of rare types which have a natural, genetic resistance, and which multiply as the non-resisters die off.

It was the awareness of this risk which inspired the World Health Organization resolution, passed in the General Assembly of 1955, which called upon the organization, in co-operation with the individual governments, for an all-out campaign, all over the world, to get rid of the malaria which mosquitoes transfer, within the six or seven years in which the insects would be liable to develop insecticide resistance. The safe deadline would be five years. Thus an all-out global attack could, in five years, rid the world of malaria, which has afflicted over 300 million people in the world and has caused over three million deaths a year.

In our time, we can see the fulfillment of the work of Laveran, Manson, Sir Ronald Ross, Surgeon-General Gorgas and Walter Reed, whose researches and lifework were directed to the conquest of insect-borne diseases, like malaria and yellow fever. Malaria can be banished from the face of the earth.

2. THE DAY TOGO SMILED

From the mountains of central Java, I received a letter and a photograph of a smiling boy. The letter said: "Do you remember the first time Togo smiled?" I did, indeed. It was an occasion which one is unlikely to forget.

We had driven our jeeps into the Hungry Hills, fording streams which had no bridges and crawling up pathless mountains to the villages of the interior. On our radiator fluttered the pennants of the United Nations Children's Fund and the World Health Organization, and our equipage included Indonesian and international doctors and *mantris,* the medical auxiliaries. They formed one of the flying columns of the war against yaws.

This is a dreadful disease which is widespread throughout the whole tropical world. It is caused by a *treponema* like that which causes syphilis, but the disease is not contracted in the same way. The micro-organism enters the body through cuts and sores and, in countries where people work in their bare feet in the fields, cuts are common and the contagion easily contracted. It afflicts every age group—from the infant at its mother's breast, getting it through mouth sores, to the old people, although "old" is a relative term when the average expectation of life is under thirty years of age. It appears as skin eruptions, the raspberry-like appearance of which accounts for its textbook name, *frambesia.* These spread into ulcers and, on the sole, cause what is known as "claw-foot," in which the foot contracts like the claw of a perching bird. But it also spreads through the body, and not only grossly disfigures that but destroys the spirit as well.

One knows when one is in a countryside ridden by yaws because it disfigures the landscape as it does the human beings. The fields are neglected, the cattle unkempt, the huts squalid, and the children miserable. The victims have no will for effort.

We drove into a village where the headman beat a gong—a hollow tree trunk—which reverberated through the hills and called the peasants to the improvised clinic. It was a pathetic gathering. Some were brought on palanquins, or carried on backs. Some crawled and others hobbled pitifully into the dusty square. One of those who crawled was Togo, a little boy.

With one shot of penicillin—about ten cents' worth—yaws can be cured. It is a modern miracle, the magnitude of which can only be realized by those who know how intractable this disease has been in the past. With one injection a doctor can transform a human life.

A week later, Togo smiled for the first time in his young life. Still a bit uncertain on his feet, he came running across the square to the clinic.

A year later, that village held a feast. It was their *Re-Birthday*—the anniversary of the disappearance of the last case of yaws. Everyone contributed; from a countryside now transformed, they brought the rice and products of a new-found energy. The women plucked the chickens. Togo shinned up the palm trees to get the coconuts. The *gamelan* band beat out dance tunes that had almost been forgotten. The old shed their years, and their memories, and frolicked with the youngsters. The local comedian mimed the walk of the claw-footed cripples and the villagers laughed—a gusty, throat-catching laugh at a remembered nightmare. The men improvised a dance in which they recalled the slow, painful sowing and harvesting of the yaws-days and, to the increasing tempo of the band, worked up to the prodigies of speed with which they could now work.

They sat down to a feast and on the mats were left untouched heaped plates, like votive offerings. They were placed for the guests who were not there—the U.N. team and the Indonesian doctors who had moved on to bring similar deliverance to thousands of villages. Within the next few years yaws can be wiped out of the tropical world.

3. JUNGLE MOLD

In 1947 a specimen of mold found in the soil of Venezuela was sent to a Yale botanist, Dr. Paul Buckholder. It seemed to have useful properties and an American pharmaceutical company took it up. The chemists isolated an active principle and crystallized it.

It had its try-out in a typhus outbreak in Bolivia, where Dr. Eugene Payne used it to treat sixteen typhus fever victims. Fifteen cases seemed hopeless, yet all rallied within twelve hours and recovered within three days.

This was repeated in an outbreak in Mexico by Dr. Joseph Smadel of the U.S. Army. The results were so striking that Dr. Smadel collected a team of army medicos and all the drug, chloromycetin, then available in the world—one pound—and flew to Malaya where an epidemic of scrub typhus was raging in the midst of a jungle war. During World War II scrub typhus had caused 25,000 casualties.

With the co-operation of the doctors of the British Colonial Service, Dr. Smadel, in March 1948, set up his unit in Kuala Lumpur. Forty cases of scrub typhus, some of them far advanced, were brought to him. The drug was administered in tablet form and, with one dose each, and within thirty-one hours, the cases had recovered. There were no failures.

The story of chloromycetin goes beyond typhus. By accident, it was found to be effective in typhoid, often confused with typhus, both in name and in the early symptoms. Typhus is louse-borne in its common form, and mite-borne in the case of scrub typhus, while typhoid is due to food or water contamination, with a bacillus.

In several cases of suspected scrub typhus, the process of the disease did not conform to normal, but Dr. Smadel persisted with the drug and effected a cure. It was then discovered that the cases were not scrub typhus but typhoid. And so yet another intransigent disease had been mastered.

4. PEACE HATH ITS VICTORIES . . .

One by one the old killer diseases are being ticked off and their names added, like chevrons to a battle standard, to the list of medical victories. And each is more momentous, though less spectacular, than the vaunted victories of our history books.

Some of my intellectual friends indulge in a parlor game called "Crossroads," in which they choose some point of departure in history and consider what would have happened if, at that crossroads, events had taken the road to the left instead of the right, or the right instead of the left—if, for instance, Lenin's sealed train had never reached Russia, or Hitler had been stopped when he entered the Rhineland. Or if Lord North had died in infancy. Perhaps some of our present-day medical achievements might be measured in their magnitude if we look at what the diseases now conquered have meant at the crossroads of history:

Alexander the Great died of malaria by the waters of Babylon in 323 B.C. in his thirty-third year. His empire stretched to the Ganges.

The Roman Empire declined, and, simultaneously, so did the enlightened Han Empire in China, in an epidemic of an ill-defined infectious disease. But we know that malaria drove the peasants off the land to crowd into the Eternal City in its decline.

The collapse of the Byzantine Empire followed the Plague of Justinian (540 A.D.) which is recognizably bubonic (which we can now successfully treat with streptomycin, of the chloramphenical or tetracycline group of antibiotics).

Syphilis, which, like its cousin, yaws, is now curable with penicillin, was probably brought to Europe by the ships of Columbus. In six years it had spread across Europe.

But Europe, in return, sent smallpox to vanquish the Aztecs. In 1520, Cortes landed at Vera Cruz with 110 mariners, 553 soldiers, 10 heavy guns and 16 horses. He occupied Tenochitlan (Mexico City), the Aztec capital, with little opposition, but he outraged the hitherto complacent Aztecs by an unnecessary massacre of the nobility. He and his forces escaped only with difficulty but his rival Narvaez had landed near Cempoalla, and in his company was a Negro slave with smallpox. It swept the land. Maxcica, King of Tlascala, died, as did Cuitlahuac, Montezuma's successor, and it was estimated that half the three and one half million inhabitants died. Cortez marched again and the Aztec Empire came to an end on August 15, 1521, eighteen months after the invasion of smallpox.

The outcome of the French Revolution was to some extent decided by dysentery (now treatable with neomycin). In 1792, Frederick William II of Prussia, with Austrian allies, and a total strength of 42,000 men marched against the armies of the Revolution. Losing 12,000 men through dysentery, the Prussians retreated across the Rhine.

Even the greatest general of all, Napoleon, was helpless against the invisible armies of infection and contagion. For his invasion of Russia, he mustered half a million men. By the time the Niemen was crossed on June 24, 1812, typhus had appeared and dysentery and enteric fever followed. He entered Moscow on September 12 and the Russians set fire to the city. When the retreat from Moscow began on October 19, there were not more than 80,000 fit for duty. By the time the stricken army reached Vilna only 20,000 remained; of Marshal Ney's crack Third Army Corps only 20 men remained. The poor vestiges of the Grande Armée were almost without exception infected with typhus.

In 1813, Napoleon raised another army of half a million men. By the time his new army faced the allies at Leipzig, it had been reduced to 170,000.

Consider how disease influenced the military history of the United States: When John Morgan took over as director general of hospitals of the Revolutionary army in 1775, he was appalled by the conditions of the army in Canada. The American colonists had taken every British stronghold except Quebec. Soon they were in full flight, attacked by dysentery, bilious fever and smallpox. His failure, because of official intrigue, to secure the proper reorganization of the army medical services to remedy this debacle, may have meant that Canada, which might have been part of the United States, survived as part of the British Commonwealth.

During the Civil War, from 1861 to 1865, 44,238 soldiers of the Federal armies were killed in battle, 49,205 died of wounds and 186,216 died of disease.

After the Revolution in Russia, twenty-five million cases of typhus were reported between 1917 and 1921 and three millions died.

Conditions of war and of the aggregations of armies have always promoted disease but consider some facts from the last war: The United States had over 2,000,000 men in North Africa, the Middle East, South East Asia and the Pacific theater—all regions where troops, with no natural immunity to tropical and pestilential diseases, were being exposed to them. Up to V-J Day, August 1945, there were no cases of plague, 241 of relapsing fever, 13 of cholera, 61 of epidemic typhus, and 7,000 cases with 300 deaths from scrub typhus, for which Smadel, two and a half years later, found the answer.

Although it is always difficult to estimate *what did not happen,* it is a conservative estimate to say that modern chemicals and drugs have, in the past ten years, saved more lives than the total casualties of the ten years of two World Wars.

Indeed, a medical statistician friend of mine, estimating for the postwar epidemics (like the pandemic of influenza in 1918-19 with 21,000,000 deaths) which should have happened and did not, claims that science, since the end of World War II, has saved more lives than have been lost in *all the wars* since *Homo sapiens,* insapiently, became belligerent.

5. BATTLE HONORS

One does not need a crystal ball to predict that, within this generation, medical science will have overcome, and controlled, all man's external enemies—the insect-borne diseases, like malaria; the parasitical diseases, like bilharzia, transmitted by a water snail; the person-to-person diseases, like yaws and syphilis; the water-, and food-, borne diseases, like the dysenteries and typhoid; the "old" pestilential diseases, like cholera, plague, smallpox, typhus, yellow fever, and leprosy; and, indeed, all infections and contagions.

In the microscopic war, the range of weapons of counterattack has now been extended to immobilize diseases for which, as recently as 1934, the doctors had no specific remedies. True they had protection by public health measures, and protection by vaccination and inoculation could, where proper health services existed, restrain the onset of the diseases. But it is rather like the Inter-Continental Ballistic Missile, about which the military talk so much today. With interception (sanitary measures), the attack might be limited. With Civil Defense (vaccination and inoculation) the effects might be reduced. But, as we know from V.1's and V.2's in World War II, some or many will always get through and the only effective answer is to strike at the bases. Before 1934, the doctors had very few weapons in their medical armory which could strike at a specific micro-organism.

Today, while we must maintain our defense systems and our Home Guard, we now possess the means to attack diseases directly. With the permutations and combinations of the sulfa and antibiotic drugs the range of attack is wide and selective. From the fungi which cause skin diseases (like athlete's foot) to the rickettsia of typhus the effectiveness of the new drugs ranges over microorganisms of diminishing size.

Beyond that spectrum still lie the small viruses, like those of influenza and polio, against which we have still to rely on protection and not on treatment, although the complications which were usually the serious accompaniment of virus diseases (like pneumonia, in influenza) can be dealt with. Again, without the crystal ball, it is possible to foresee the time when the answer will similarly be found to the viruses. And when it is we shall be getting critically near the heart of all living nature, for the virus is smaller than the living cell itself and capable of penetrating it and the drug will have to kill the virus without damaging the cell.

In the meantime, while we are waiting for the means of direct attack against viruses, immunology can provide community defenses by measures such as the Salk vaccine. Such preventive measures may themselves reduce a disease to relative insignificance, as the world has seen through vaccination against smallpox and prophylactic inoculation against diphtheria. In fact we can return to Virchow's analogy of the "sick state" and the "sick body." When an infection invades the body the natural defenders, the antibodies, mobilize to repel it. If the disease is virulent, it will overwhelm the defenses before they are adequately prepared and the illness will follow. If, however, the infection is mild then the muster of antibodies will arrest the germs, as militiamen might "pick up" paratroopers (although they could not repel a task force). But, once the body-militia have been fully alerted, they remain organized to resist a more massive infection. The presence even of a dead virus, as in the case of the Salk polio vaccine, brings about an effective mobilization.

In large, that is true of the community itself. If a disease is in serious proportion, then the public health services will find it hard to bring it under control. But once immunization has reduced the outbreaks to sporadic cases those "antibodies" of the community, the medical officers of health, can deal with the infection, isolate it and treat it, so that it is no longer a menace.

Even truculent diseases, like tuberculosis, "the White

Plague," once the world's biggest killer, are now coming under control. Tuberculosis is a community disease, that is to say, it is communicated by close contact and exaggerated by conditions of living—bad housing, overcrowding and undernourishment. The only answer until a few years ago was to segregate the active cases in sanatoria and, by long rest and good food and good air, to give nature a chance to resist the infection. The surgeons could help by operations. By isolating cases, to protect the rest of the community, and by slow improvement of the conditions which we know encourage the disease, society might gradually have won a Thirty Years' War.

Now we have other means. Hundreds of millions of people have been given an artificial protection against the disease by B.C.G. (Bacillus-Calmette-Guerin). This is a live vaccine, which means that a very mild strain of tuberculosis is injected to mobilize the body against further infection. After the war, when the ravages and the displacements of millions of people might have led to a flaming outbreak of tuberculosis throughout the world, first UNRRA (the United Nations Relief and Rehabilitation Administration) and later UNICEF (the United Nations Children's Fund) undertook wholesale inoculation with B.C.G. The campaign still goes on, and the benefits are immeasurable, because, once again, we cannot measure what has not happened—the deaths that might have occurred.

Then it was found that *streptomycin,* the antibiotic discovered by Dr. Selman Waksman, of Rutgers University, New Jersey, in 1944, could destroy the tubercule bacillus in test tubes and check active tuberculosis in mice. After a period of the usual overoptimism, and consequent disappointment, the antibiotic has taken its permanent place in treatment of tuberculosis but usually in conjunction with P.A.S. (*Para-Amino-Salicylic acid*) or *isoniazid,* two "tailor-made" drugs. As a result of these new drugs active tuberculosis is at last being got under control.

I have seen the interesting effects of the chemists' intervention among the Eskimos, in the Arctic. Tuberculosis was gaining ground and looked as though it might eventually wipe out the race. The doctors would tour the Arctic and find the active cases and would try to remove them to sanatoria in the south, to prevent them from infecting others. The Eskimos are an amenable people but they could not help noticing that few who went south ever came back, which was poor encouragement to others. There were always liable to be hidden cases, spreading the disease. Nowadays with antibiotics and chemical drugs, deaths in the south are becoming more and more rare and Eskimos are returning to the Arctic cured. Today, getting into a plane with a tuberculosis ticket has become an adventure for the Eskimo, who can count on booking a round trip. The result is they are ready and willing to go and, by their going, sources of infection are removed. Thus successful treatment helps prevention and tuberculosis is disappearing from the Arctic. Out of 900 Eskimos examined by a Flying Clinic which I joined in the Arctic, not a single new case of tuberculosis was discovered.

Treatment is never a substitute for prevention and, in diseases like tuberculosis, the short cuts must not discourage the social measures to remove the conditions in which the disease is fostered, nor replace the conservative treatment which builds up resistant bodies.

6. ARC DE TRIOMPHE

If we were playing that game "Crossroads" in terms of the points of departure in the progress against the germs, man's external enemies, it would be like standing on the Arc de Triomphe in the center of the Etoile, in Paris, with the roads branching out in every direction, but the avenues would carry the names not of generals and battles but of discoverers.

Avenue Leeuwenhoek would recall the son of a basketmaker, born in 1632 in Delft, Holland. It was he who first used the Janssen "flea-glasses" to observe "little animals." He was the first to observe protozoa, and the human male sperm, as well as bacteria and disease bacilli. He discovered that rain water, after contact with city atmosphere, was alive with little animals ten thousand times smaller than the water fleas which could be observed with the naked eye.

In the famous "Letter 18" written to the Royal Society of London, he described "a sort of little animal, incredibly small. Nay, so small, in my sight, that I judged that even if one hundred of these very tiny animals lay stretched out one against another, they could not reach the length of a grain of coarse sand and ten hundred thousand of these living creatures would scarce equal the bulk of a coarse grain of sand."

He took scrapings of his teeth and, not having the advantages of the modern microscopic camera, he drew, recognizably even today, the germs which he found in his mouth and studied under the microscope.

"How be it," he asked, "that I clean my mouth yet all the people living in our united Netherlands are not as many as the living animals I carry in my own mouth on this very day?"

Avenue Virchow would recognize the German who made the disease processes in the body intelligible and explain how they were upset by "external forces."

Avenue Pasteur would replace the *Avenue Grande Armée,* that majestic boulevard of Paris, if we could rename it, in honor of a man who was greater, to the glory of France, then the Grande Armée itself. Louis Pasteur (1822-95) was the son of a Sergeant Major in that army. In 1857, while a professor at Lille, he was confronted with a practical problem. A key industry, which made alcohol from beetroot, was in a bad way and he was asked for his advice. So began the eventful study of the life cycle of yeast cells, in the various brews sent to him by the distillers.

Until then it had been generally accepted that fermentation was a purely chemical action resulting from the chemical breakdown of dead yeast. Pasteur proved the opposite—that fermentation was a living process. He showed that yeast organisms, fed on some sugary liquid and *exposed to air* absorb oxygen, multiply rapidly and produce very little alcohol, but when yeast organisms are placed in a sugary solution *without air,* they produce alcohol in large quantities. In short, yeast, which, in order to live, needs oxygen, can get it easily from the air, and will do so if air is available, but if it cannot get its oxygen any other way it will break down the sugar to get the oxygen from it and will leave alcohol, which is sugar without oxygen.

Pasteur went on to show that vinegar is similarly produced in the decomposition of wine and that butyric acid is produced in rancid butter. This is the process which we call "fermentation" when we find it useful and "putrefaction" when we do not want it. He was able to culture his micro-organisms, and, under the artificial conditions on which scientists insist, was able to demonstrate over and over again that there would be no decay of any tissues except by oxidation if it were not for these tiny living organisms. In other words, a piece of flesh would shrivel but it would not putrefy if there were no micro-organisms in the atmosphere.

He went on to destroy forever the idea of "spontaneous generation," a tenet held by classical scientists ever since Aristotle. He took twenty flasks of broth up into the Alps into the pure atmosphere and opened them to the air, and only one, probably previously infected, showed any decomposition. Even the French Academy had then to accept Pasteur's conclusion "that germs have parents like men themselves." To his fundamental discoveries he added the practical discoveries of vaccines against anthrax and against rabies.

Avenue Semmelweis would recall Ignaz Semmelweis (1818-65), a Hungarian who became an assistant in the maternity wards of the Vienna General Hospital. For a mother to be taken to one ward was almost certain death. It was so notorious that women begged with tears to be spared going into it. In a second ward, the death rate was not so high, and Semmelweis noted that the difference between the two was that the first was used for midwifery demonstrations to medical students who came from the dissecting room and handled the cases without bothering even to wash their hands. The second ward was used for the instruction of midwives, who had not handled cadavers and had better standards of cleanliness. This struck Semmelweis forcibly and he began to make systematic post-mortem examinations of fatal childbirth cases. Then one of his colleagues died as a result of cutting himself in dissecting a corpse from the General Hospital; Semmelweis attended the post-mortem. He noticed the similarity between the condition of his friend and the pathological appearance of his childbed cases. He was convinced, and, in his own ward, established rigorous conditions of cleanliness, with the result that within a year, instead of one in ten of the mothers dying, he got it down to four in a hundred.

In the next year he had reduced it to 1.27 per cent, and all by the simple expedient of washing the hands in chloride of lime before assisting at a birth.

He encountered the same violent reaction from his colleagues as Oliver Wendell Holmes had encountered in the United States, when, from independent observation, he had insisted that doctors should wash their hands in chloride of lime. (Holmes did not lessen the opposition of his American colleagues when he invoked Semmelweis in support of his argument.) But the Hungarian did not have the self-assurance of the Autocrat at the Breakfast-Table and the persecution drove him insane, even while Pasteur's discoveries were proving how right he was.

Avenue Lister would be next to *Avenue Pasteur,* because Joseph, Lord Lister (1827-1912) was Pasteur's greatest ally.

He was born at Upton House, in Essex, the son of a Quaker merchant. He became a student of surgery in those days when J. Y. Simpson, of chloroform fame, said: "A man laid on the operating table of one of our surgical hospitals is exposed to more chances of death than a soldier on the battlefield of Waterloo." Surgery meant unspeakable agonies and nearly half of the cases died through septic poisoning and "hospital diseases."

In 1865, when Lister was professor of Surgery at Glasgow University, his attention was drawn by his colleague in the chair of chemistry to the proceedings of the French Academy and to the accounts there of Pasteur's work emphasizing that putrefactions were caused by living ferments. Lister immediately recognized the medical applications of this, if it were true. Observation persuaded him that inflammation, suppuration of wounds, and sepsis in surgical patients, were indeed living processes, in the service of Death. He first tried using zinc chloride as an antiseptic, without much success, and then he heard that the city of Carlisle had successfully used carbolic acid in the disinfection of sewage.

That was the beginning of antisepsis. Lister used a carbolic acid spray to prevent the infection of wounds during operations. He was (as always with medical pioneers) derided by his colleagues, but his recoveries compared so conspicuously well with their losses that his example prevailed. Surgery, which had been confined almost entirely to amputations—and then with only half a chance of survival—could now be extended, by antisepsis and rigorous cleanliness, to internal surgery. Today *anti*-sepsis has been replaced in hospital practice by *a*-sepsis: in-

stead of killing the germs when they attack a fresh, or
surgical, wound everything conceivable—air conditioning, sterilization, germicidal lamps and immaculate cleanliness in the human personnel—is done to ensure that
germs never get near the wounds at all. Asepsis accepts
Pasteur's contention that the flesh would not putrefy in an
atmosphere entirely free from micro-organisms. (And,
here, one might, with good grace, recall Rhases, the Lute
Player of Baghdad, recorded earlier in this book, who,
more than a thousand years before Pasteur, hung up meat
in various parts of the city and chose, as the site of
the Caliph's hospital, the part where the meat putrefied
least. If Rhases cannot have an avenue, he might have
a cul-de-sac.)

Avenue Koch would be where *Avenue Foch* is. Robert
Koch (1843-1910) was the local doctor in the little town
of Wollstein, Germany. He was a self-taught bacteriologist, but his techniques of research were what scientists
call "beautiful." He set himself to study the life history
of the anthrax bacillus. His method illustrates the true
scientific approach. He found the bacillus in the blood,
spleen and elsewhere in the body of an animal dead of
anthrax. He cultivated the bacillus in blood serum and in
the fluid from the eye of an ox. He studied the cultures
he thus made and observed every stage of the growth of
the bacillus, the propagation of spores, and, removing
those spores to fresh cultures, watched them grow into
bacilli.

From those test-tube cultures he produced anthrax in a
mouse, and transferred it from mouse to mouse in a long
series. Then from the last mouse he obtained a bacillus
from which to breed a new culture. And this he did,
over and over again, proving to his own satisfaction that
the anthrax "bred true." This was the first germ proved
to be causative of a disease in man.

He proceeded to isolate and test by such methods the
bacillus of tuberculosis and the vibrio of cholera. He was
the standard bearer at the head of that long procession
of systematic bacteriologists which extends to the present day.

Avenue Ehrlich would be next to that of his colleague
Koch.

Paul Ehrlich (1854-1915) became Koch's assistant.
He was the son of a Jewish tradesman born in Strehlen,

Silesia. He was definitely a "late developer." At school he was a dunderhead and his professors at the university concurred with his schoolmasters. He failed in his finals, which was scarcely surprising, because he had an aversion to lectures and preferred to potter around the chemical laboratory, fiddling with dyes. When Koch went to Breslau to demonstrate his anthrax bacillus, the professors tried to hurry him past an untidy corner in the barrack-prim laboratory; it was Ehrlich's littered, dye-stained bench.

At last, he qualified in medicine and went on to his doctorate. Then the unpredictable Ehrlich startled everyone by his brilliant thesis on the coloring of histological tissue—that is, the thin sections of tissue with the cells differentially dyed to distinguish them under the microscope, a technique employed by Koch.

Ehrlich had, in that untidy corner, been studying the symptoms of lead poisoning in rabbits and he noticed that those organs which had been worst affected in the living body also had an affinity to lead after death. This led him to conclude that certain minerals and dyes had a special liking for certain tissues and that this affinity could be used to study the organic effects of bacterial disease.

But his momentous contribution was his realization that if cells and tissues had a way of selecting dyes, dyes could be used as express messengers to carry special deliveries to any part of the body. For example, when he injected methylene blue into an animal he found that only the nerves of the animal and no other tissue was stained. Perhaps, he argued, it would be possible to provide methylene blue with a chemical knapsack—attach a fraction of narcotic to the dye and ensure that it would be delivered to the nervous system to deaden pain. He also argued that it should be possible to inject into the living body specific dyes which would seek out, not only specific tissues, but specific germs. Hence Ehrlich's 606, or salvarsan, the "magic bullet" which he found, after 606 experiments, would "home in" on the spirochete of syphilis *within the body*. That is the important thing— *within the body*. Antiseptics could kill germs if they could reach them on the surface, but the carbolic acid which would kill a germ in a flesh wound would kill the patient if he drank it. Now here, thanks to Ehrlich, was a veritable Daniel Boone of an antiseptic, tracking through the body, to snipe the spirochete.

Avenue Jenner would replace *Avenue Jena* to commemorate the man who introduced vaccination as a Western medical practice.

And there ought to be an *Avenue Theobald Smith* (1859-1934) to honor the Harvard professor of pathology who first demonstrated immunization, as distinct from vaccination.

In 1886, working with D. E. Salmon, he showed that the introduction of dead microbes into the body led to the development of immunity. In this case it was the bacillus of hog cholera. If it was injected into a pigeon, it killed the bird, but if the germs were killed by heat first, it created a resistance to a dose of the living microbe.

This was the beginning of the understanding of immunology, which today is a very important science, with a meaning beyond the reactions to germs. It explains how the body produces antibodies—substances which deal with any intruder substances foreign to the body (antigens) in ways specific to each. They will deal in one way with toxins; in another with germs, dissolving them, or making them easier for the white blood cells to overcome. They explain some of the allergies—pollen produces in some people a violent "immunological" response which we call hay fever. They account for the risks in blood transfusion and why such care has to be taken in giving the right blood group because the wrong one would produce antibodies which would make the patient's blood cells clump, or agglutinate. This xenophobia, or rejection of alien cells, also accounts for the fact that a skin graft from another person (unless it is an identical twin) will not "take" and will simply scale off, because the antibodies discard cells which have not the identical genes, or hereditary factors.

But at the end of the nineteenth century, Theobald Smith's contribution helped doctors to understand better the fourfold defense of the body against invading germs: First, there is the germproof skin, adequate until a cut or sore provides a gateway. Secondly, there are the white cells, the leucocytes, which rally to repel invaders through such portals; the pus which forms on a festering wound is made up of the corpses of leucocytes which have tried to block the invaders. Thirdly, there is the heat resistance;

when germs are in force the heat of the body rises (the fever) to weaken the micro-organisms and assist the other defenses. Fourthly, there are the antibodies.

Avenue Domagk would symbolize another new departure. Gerhard Domagk was the bacteriologist of the I. G. Farben chemical combine in Germany who initiated the era of the sulfa drugs. That was in 1934, but back in 1908, seven years before Ehrlich's death, a young Austrian, Paul Gelmo, submitted a thesis for his doctorate at the Vienna Institute of Technology. He had synthesized a new coal-tar derivative which he called "para-amino-benzene-sulfonamide." He did not patent it but described it and stepped out of history until, after the second World War, he was found modestly working as a chemist for an Austrian printing firm.

I. G. Farben discovered Gelmo's sulfonamide in the dyestuff literature. At first, it was thought of merely as a possible dye for textiles, but Domagk was following up the work of Ehrlich and trying to find a good germicide which would kill germs, as *salvarsan* does, within the living body. In 1932, a red dye in which Domagk saw promising possibilities was produced and patented. He infected literally thousands of mice with streptococcal infection, which should have killed them all within three days. With the red dye, *prontosil,* they survived.

Then there was a dramatic denouement. Domagk was still unsure of the effects on humans, when his own daughter contracted a virulent streptococcal infection from the prick of a knitting needle and generalized blood poisoning set in. The doctors and surgeons despaired of her life. Her desperate father took the risk—he administered a large dose of prontosil. She recovered completely. But he was a good scientist; he would make no claim on one case; it would not be statistically significant; and instead, when he reported on experimental evidence for prontosil he mentioned only his mice experiments.

In 1936, the confirmation came on a sufficient scale. Dr. Leonard Colebrook at Queen Charlotte's Hospital, the London maternity institution, was faced with thirty-eight cases of mothers with deadly childbirth fever. On past experience, one in four would certainly die. They tried prontosil: only three died. The next series was even better and prontosil "hit the headlines" and the Miracle Drugs were with us. Ehrlich rode again and the medical and scientific world were reminded of his principle that drugs could be found to kill germs within the body.

Avenue Fleming would be the Champs Elysées of our bacteriological Arch of Triumph, of our chemotherapeutic Etoile, although it should be a three-lane boulevard because the Nobel Prize for penicillin was shared by Sir Alexander Fleming, Sir Howard Florey and Dr. Ernest Chain.

To the story books of all time belongs the incident at St. Mary's Hospital, alongside London's Paddington Station, one morning in September 1928. Professor Fleming had been on vacation but before setting out he had left a variety of germs to breed in shallow dishes with glass lids, and now he was inspecting the dishes to see how the colonies had multiplied.

The lid of one, on a window ledge, had slipped. Fleming examined it. It had been "spoiled" because a mold had come in through the window, out of dusty London, and had settled on it. Before he threw it into the garbage pail, Fleming had a second look. That hesitation changed medical history.

What he saw excited Fleming. He was a trained bacteriologist and a superb laboratory technician and the discoverer of *lysozyme,* the factor in the tears which dissolves, and protects our eyes against, the germs which are everywhere in our atmosphere. It was the awareness of "lysis" which made him pause.

Around the bit of fluff, that mold, was a clear moat dividing it from the colony of germs which had proliferated all around. It struck Fleming that the mold might be exuding some substance which was acting like *lysozyme*. He cultivated that mold and, from the broth on which he fed it, tried to isolate the substance. It "worked" on germs in test tubes and in culture dishes and he found that it worked on some germs and not on others and so acted as a laboratory "scavenger" killing off unwanted germs in certain cultures. He tried it on surface infections, like sties and boils, and it worked. But it was what chemists call "labile," or unstable; it lost its effectiveness very quickly and was unreliable. And long-tried antiseptics were less trouble for surface use. (Notice, he had not thought of it for killing germs *within the body*.)

And penicillin, in which Fleming as a bacteriologist believed, but which he could not make biochemically effective, remained a laboratory curiosity until 1938. Then Ernest Chain, a refugee from Germany, working with Professor Howard Florey at Oxford University, came upon the records by accident. He was, with Florey, re-examining Fleming's original ideas about the tear-factor and chanced upon the penicillin papers in the Radcliffe Library at Oxford. But the thing which had discouraged Fleming—the instability of the penicillin secretion—was what intrigued Chain, the biochemist. And he and his chief both realized that here was a germicide which might act benevolently *within the body*. Why should it occur to them in 1938 and not to Fleming, in 1928? Because the sulfa drugs had changed the scientific climate and doctors were again "inward-minded," as Ehrlich had been.

The result was the epoch-making discovery of the penicillin drug as we know it today, forerunner of that procession of antibiotics. Fleming had discovered the effect, Chain had "spotted" the chemistry, and Florey had foreseen and applied the clinical advantages.

The first clinical trial was a desperate one. On February 12, 1941, it was administered to a police constable who was suffering from a generalized blood poisoning, due to an unholy alliance between streptococci and staphylococci. The sulfa drugs having been tried without success the patient's life was despaired of. Penicillin was administered as a last resort. The improvement was immediate and after two days he was recovering. But the supplies of the drug gave out. He relapsed and died.

There was no doubt, however, that the drug showed every promise. The first problem was availability of supplies and the second was to see that the body retained enough of it to act on the germs—it was excreted too quickly. The first was a matter of time; the second, until more powerful and slower acting versions of the drug were obtained, was overcome by dripping liquid penicillin into the veins.

The first time that Fleming handled the powder which had eluded him since 1929 was on August 6, 1942. A personal friend was dying of meningitis, caused by a germ which Fleming himself had shown to be susceptible to penicillin. The patient was surely dying. Fleming asked Florey for help and Florey took the entire supply of penicillin then available in Britain to St. Mary's Hospital, where Fleming himself injected the drug into the muscle and later into the spine. Three weeks later the patient was allowed out of bed. A month later he left the hospital completely cured.

Where all these avenues meet at the crossroads would stand the triumphal arch which celebrates the victories over the external enemies, the micro-organisms, and under that arch would burn the deathless flame by which we remember the many others who worked and died to free the world from pestilence. And we should inscribe for them the epitaph of Lazear, member of the American Commission led by Walter Reed to fight yellow fever in Cuba. Lazear submitted to being bitten by a mosquito which had fed on yellow-fever cases and he died of it. Of him it was said:

"With more than the courage and devotion of a soldier, he risked and lost his life to show how a fearful pestilence is communicated and how its ravages can be prevented."

Part Eleven

UNFINISHED BUSINESS

> I took a life, and the only way I can
> atone for that, even in a small measure,
> is through something like cancer re-
> search.
>
> —Letter from a condemned murderer
> to Mr. Ralph Alvis, Warden of Ohio
> Penitentiary. (Quoted by *Time* Maga-
> zine)

1. DEATH CELL

In the eyes of the law, the convicts in Ohio penitentiary,
Columbus, were a tough lot—killers in for life, bank
robbers and men of violence. When, however, volunteers
were called for to expose themselves to a cancer experiment, 150 responded and 53 were chosen. For the benefit of others, they were prepared to become human guinea
pigs and submit to inoculations of malignant disease.
They were prepared to accept the "death cell" as an injection into their bodies.

Under heavy guard, the volunteers paraded and
waited their turn. As each man's name was called he entered the surgery improvised in the prison by Dr. Chester
M. Southam, of the Sloan-Kettering Institute, New York.
Each convict exposed his arm.

Malignant cells from human victims of the disease had
been cultivated at the Institute. First, a patch of the arm
about three inches in diameter was anesthetized. In the
center Dr. Southam stuck a tattoo needle, to provide a
permanent reference mark. Then filling a hypodermic
syringe with three and a half million cancer cells, he injected them under the skin. Lower down the arm he gave
a second injection of the same amount. Into the arms
of some of them he transplanted tissues of other cancer
strains, artificially cultivated.

The aim was to discover whether a healthy individual—
and all the convicts, including the "lifers" selected, were

215

first-class "lifes"—had an immunity to implanted cancer. In advanced cases of cancer this mechanism of rejection seems to be absent. This test might throw an interesting light on the disease, because, as we have seen earlier in this book, the body resists and rejects the cells of other people. (That is why cells of the wrong blood group cause serious complications in transfusion and why a skin graft from someone else will not "take" but will simply slough.)

In a matter of hours or days some of the injection sites swelled up and became inflamed. This was the healthy body's natural reaction; the defenses were disposing of the invaders. In other cases the volunteers had no discomfort at all; the swelling just disappeared; again there was no cause for medical concern because the body defenses had disposed of the cancer cells without any difficulty.

Three weeks later, a surgeon measured an inch and half below the tattoo mark in each case and opened the arm and removed the tissue which had embraced the implanted cells. In some cases it was found that all the cancer cells had disappeared. It was also found that implants which were not surgically removed in this way, had disappeared within a month.

This research was reassuring as showing the immunity reaction, to cancer, of healthy subjects. None of the convicts contracted, or is likely to contract, the disease as a result of the experiment. That, however, does not diminish the courage of the convict-volunteers who thus submitted to the first experiment in transferring cancer. And, indeed, they are the more praiseworthy because this was a piece of pure research and not something which could be applied directly to the treatment of cancer victims.

2. WHAT IS CANCER?

This episode was just another incident in the intensive quest to find the answer to one of the most baffling puzzles of nature: How do normal cells become anarchical and produce malignant disease, within the body?

One of the difficulties, particularly in popular understanding, is the idea that cancer is a specific disease. To say that someone "died of cancer" is like saying, a hundred years ago, "He died of a fever." Today, we know that a fever may be due to any one of the vast array of micro-organisms. A "fever" is not a cause of death; it is a symptom of a process. So is cancer.

As Virchow showed, a cell that causes a disease condition is not a sickly cell but on the contrary a robust one. The cell in a malignant growth is like a powerful bully: it grabs, greedily, the chemical foods on which cells live; it waxes strong and propagates faster than the surrounding cells. It is a cuckoo in the nest. The result is to destroy the normal tissue and to cause that condition which we call "cancer." A cancer, therefore, is an abnormal proliferation of cells.

If the teeming cells are localized and are accessible to the surgeon's knife, to radiations, or to the modern radioactive isotopes, the abnormal cells can be cut out or killed to give the normal cells a fair chance. Surgery in recent years has had encouraging, and numerous, successes in thus arresting cancer—if the cases can be detected in time. That is the rub—like Attila's Huns, and Hitler's Nazis, abnormal cells seek *lebensraum;* they migrate to spread disruption elsewhere. They spread, like *panzer* columns, through the blood and the lymph streams and establish colonies in various parts of the body. They infiltrate and choke vital organs and destroy the processes on which life depends.

With the best will in the world, and with the finest resources, the *surgeons* can never provide the ultimate answer to cancer. They can try, often with success, to eradicate the "seeds" of cancer. But if the seeds break loose, the surgeon cannot track them all. The answer, therefore, must be found in a different approach. Just as we have found specific drugs to kill specific germs so medical science must find a means of dealing with specific cancer cells within specific sites of the body. Already they know that sex hormones have an effect on certain forms of cancer—in the prostate gland and in the breasts, they can inhibit the growth and spread of the abnormal cells.

In many diseases, the cure has been found before the cause, but in cancer—in all its variations—the desperately sought-for answers may have to await the full understanding, still elusive, of the fundamentals of the process. Because the abnormal is bound up with the normal this is difficult—but it is not beyond the wit of man.

The process is involved with genetics, the study of the

characteristics of the cells which are transmitted from generation to generation. This does not mean that cancer itself is necessarily inherited, as is the case with diseases like hemophilia, in which the blood fails to clot. Heredity may account for a predisposition to cancer, without the disease itself being transmitted. Our cells all derive from the cells of our parents and of our ancestors. They "organize" themselves to give us those recognizable resemblances—the color of the hair and the eyes, the shape of the nose, our father's height, our mother's temperament, etc. Within the body individual cells also pass on their hereditary factors through the *chromosomes,* or packages of *genes*. More specifically it is a particular chemical within the *chromosomes*—deoxyribonucleic acid (DNA, for short)—which decides the characteristics. So, according to the most plausible theory of today, a cell becomes cancerous either when something happens to the structure of its nucleic acid or to the way the cell acquires and uses the chemicals of the body.

3. DNA

The clue to cancer, therefore, may lie in DNA, this fundamental chemical of life. Sir Alexander Todd, the biochemist; Dr. F. H. C. Crick and the American Professor J. D. Watson, two physicists working at the Cambridge Laboratory; and Dr. M. F. H. Wilkins, of King's College, London, carried out researches into the structure of DNA, chemically and physically. By X-rays it was possible to show how the atoms of the individual elements were arranged in the nucleic acid. They were able to produce a model of a spiral or helical molecule and from its structure to suggest how a chemical of this kind could reproduce itself—"live," in fact; how it would attract and select the elements from the chemical medium around it. Cancerous cells apparently produce more nucleic acid than normal ones do. They also apparently have their own characteristic patterns of manufacture and may use a certain element or elements in greater amounts at particular stages.

Here is a definite lead. We have the analogy of the sulfa drugs which destroy bacteria because they substitute for a chemical indispensable to the survival of the bacteria, another chemical which the bacteria will accept but which will be useless to it. With the substitute chemical it will not reproduce itself. Since the abnormal cells of cancer have an addiction to certain chemicals which normal cells have not, it ought to be possible to replace those chemicals by bogus ones, so that the cancer cell, in its greed and gluttony, will die and the ordinary cells survive.

There are already proofs of this possibility. One of the basic chemicals of the body is *folic acid,* which the cells of the blood cancer, *leukemia,* require in greater amounts than normal cells. In the same chemical "family" as folic acid (*pterygoglutamic acid*) is *aminopterin,* which cancer cells will accept in place of the other but which will prevent their growth.

4. BUTTERFLY WINGS

Notice the words "pterygoglutamic" and "aminopterin," and, especially, the "pterin." That comes from the Greek word meaning "wing." And thereby hangs one of the delightful, human stories of science.

When Dr. Tom Spies, in the U.S.A., discovered the values of folic acid in the treatment of the tropical disease, sprue, I, in London, had to find out something about it. I was on my way to the Royal Society, in Piccadilly, to make the inquiry and, dodging my way in the traffic of that thoroughfare, I found myself marooned on an island with Sir Robert Robinson, the Nobel Prize-winning chemist and then president of the Royal. Above the roar of the traffic I shouted "Tell me, What is folic acid?" and he shouted back "Surely you know! It's Hoppy's butterfly wings."

"Hoppy" was Sir Frederick Gowland Hopkins, pioneer of vitamins, Nobel Prize-winner, member of that rare company, Britain's Order of Merit, president of the Royal Society, president of the British Association, etc., etc., etc.

Time was when he was a lonely little boy chasing butterflies around the hedgerows of Middlesex on the outskirts of London. He was fascinated by butterflies, moths and beetles. His father was dead and an unsympathetic uncle, ignoring his scientific urge, sent him into an insurance office. There, still chasing his insects, he wrote a paper on the bombardier beetle, describing how when it was disturbed it injected a violet vapor into the air and how he had collected some of this in a test tube and had tried to analyze it. And he sent the paper —his first—to *The Entomologist*.

In later years he wrote: "From that time my fate was sealed; although the designation had not yet been invented, I became there and then a biochemist at heart."

A small inheritance enabled him to escape from the insurance world and to take up science. And he still kept his interest in butterflies. In 1889, at the age of twenty-eight, having "learned his trade," he started to work on the pigment of butterfly wings. In 1896, while he was working at Guy's Hospital as an assistant to a specialist in forensic medicine and helping to solve some of the great murder mysteries of his time, he took time off to present a paper to the Royal Society on the pigments of butterfly wings. He showed that the opaque white of butterfly wings was uric acid and that the yellow of the wing was a related substance which could be produced when uric acid is heated under pressure. At that moment he was very near a great discovery but he had not then the refined methods of which he became the master. He made many outstanding discoveries and had honors heaped upon him—but he never forgot his butterflies. "Why doesn't Hoppy forget this butterfly foolishness?" I remember one of his august colleagues saying to me when Gowland Hopkins was in his seventies.

When he was eighty and too blind to see the color of butterfly wings, he delivered the last paper of his career to the Royal Society; it was on "pterins"—butterfly wings. But by then they had acquired a completely new significance. It had been found that the pigments were not simple uric acid derivatives, but formed a group of exciting compounds (dutifully called "pterins") which were at the very roots of life, of vitamins, of cancer-causing and cancer-inhibiting agencies, and of the pyramadine group in nucleic acid of the cell.

Hoppy was the Eternal Boy—the scientist who will chase a will-o'-the-wisp and prove it to be CH_4, or chase a butterfly through the hedgerows and into the heart of the living cell.

5. SMOKING AND CANCER

When one says such-and-such "causes" cancer, what is meant is that it triggers off that process which we still imperfectly understand.

For example, no scientist nowadays would dispute the statistical evidence that there is a correlation between smoking and lung cancer, and smokers, and those who promote smoking, though they may protest at, or ignore, the warnings had best accept the inescapable truth. That does not mean that those who do not smoke will escape lung cancer, nor that everyone who smokes cigarettes in excess will inevitably get it—any more than clay-pipe smokers will inevitably get lip cancer, though some of them have. What it means is that those of us who persist are increasing the risk that cigarettes may trigger off a disposition in our lung cells towards abnormality. It has been argued, for example, that the urge to heavy cigarette smoking may itself be a temperamental sign of a constitutional weakness which might be susceptible to cancer irritation.

Research ought presently to show what the actual cancer-inciting factor is in the cigarette (since cigar- and pipe-smokers are less liable, statistically), but when it does it will have explained no more than the specific irritation—just like saying that tar or croton oil "causes" chimney sweeps' and spinners' cancer. But that will not explain the mechanism by which it triggers off the normal living cell, the unit of life from which the body is compounded, to run riot and grow independent, to act as a Fifth Column in Virchow's "body state."

There will be many part answers and much substantial progress in the methods, surgical and medical, of treating the disease. Chemotherapeutic substances may do against disease cells what the sulfas and antibiotics have done against the germs. Enormous sums of money, especially in America, from government and private sources, are being expended on this kind of research—testing every conceivable kind of chemical compound, hormones, insecticides, weed-killers, everything. Physicists, already the allies of the surgeons, through X rays, radium and radioisotopes, are helping the geneticists to explain how deep X rays, for example, can break the atomic bonds of a chromosome in a cell to kill—or cause—a cancer; how the radiations from nuclear bombs can create leukemia (blood cancer) or cause mutations in the hereditary characteristics of a cell; and what conceivable connection there can be between mustard gas and Marie Curie's radium, yet both affect abnormal cells; or between "cobalt bombs" and "butterfly wings" or ultraviolet light and the hormones of the sex glands.

Here, in the microscopic bridgehead of life, the task forces of all the branches of science are converging. When they breach the West Wall of cancer, they will be invading the secret hinterland of Life itself.

6. "AS OLD AS HIS ARTERIES"

It has been said: "A man is as old as his arteries," and the cynic has added: "A woman is as old as her glands."

As age advances, the body—having survived the onslaught of germs, the whims of nutrition which we call "diet," the near-miss of a passing automobile, and all the other hazards of modern civilization—begins to change, and for no more reason than the passage of time. That span in which growing up and maturing becomes aging and ultimately senility varies not only from individual to individual but also from family to family. The signs are not chronological. With age, hair turns gray (but some may grow gray in their twenties); the hair wears thin and is not replaced (but baldness, which is common in advanced years, is not peculiar to them); the skin becomes less elastic and "leathery," but creasing and wrinkling do not carry a date-line; the eyes begin to fail, but "spectacles on nose" are no longer confined to the "lean and slippered pantaloon," nor hearing aids to old gaffers. Joints get stiff, but there can be nimble men of seventy and arthritics of thirty.

In women, the phase between puberty and the climacteric is fairly well defined by the capacity for childbearing, but that span can also vary between individuals and certainly between races. That is why the physiologist might agree that "a woman is as old as her glands." In men the changes are less specifically defined—like aged Justice Holmes admiring a young girl and sighing: "I wish I were eighty again"—and in them change is reflected mainly in the blood vessels, the heart, the lungs and the nervous system. Again the physiologist would agree with the saying that: "A man is as old as his arteries."

The body is like an automobile tire. The life of a tire depends on the quality of the original rubber and the make, but it also depends on how far and how fast it is driven, how many corners it has skidded round and how many punctures (traumata) it has suffered on the way. It will eventually degenerate with age—even if it is not driven at all. So with the human body. We speak of a "well-preserved old gentleman." That means he inherited a good constitution and made a good start on life's highway; that he traveled far, but not too fast, had not cut too many corners, and had not had too many "blowouts."

What are called the "degenerative diseases" are inherent in the process of aging, but frequently they get out of time-phase. For example, diabetes would be understandable if it were a case of the Islets of Langerhans giving out at the end of their working life, but it affects all ages, nowadays. And we do not know what causes it. Failure of the Islets, yes, but how and why?

So, too, with vascular diseases—failures of the blood vessels. Arteries are muscular tubes, partially constricted to maintain a pressure through the heart-pump necessary to get the blood up to the head against gravity. The muscles of the tubes also have to relax periodically to pass through different quantities of blood to meet the needs of the organs which they supply. The action of the artery muscles is, like that of the heart muscles, continuous, and the inner coats of the arteries are continuously exposed to the full pressure of the blood.

No wonder the arteries wear out in time. The degenerative process starts in the inner coat. Sometimes it is clogged with a deposition of fat, "furring" the tube as kitchen grease would gradually clog a waste pipe. (And chemists would like to find a really effective and harmless blood detergent which would remove this fatty deposit.) This obstructs the flow in the smaller arteries. Sometimes the inner coating gets roughened and, if the blood clings, clots may form, building up a log jam in the blood stream, or breaking loose to form, perhaps, a blockage in the vessels of the heart or brain, which may be fatal as a coronary or cerebral thrombosis. Progressive degeneration then spreads to the muscular coat, and the elastic tissue is replaced by fibrous tissue and sometimes by deposits of calcium salts so that the flexible tube becomes an intractable pipe. Then it is called "arteriosclerosis" or "hardening of the arteries." The rigid tube cannot accommodate itself to the varying demands of the organ it serves.

If this thickening or hardening affects the main arteries additional demands are made on the heart. Without the co-operation of the muscles of the arteries, the heart has to increase the pressure. High blood pressure is the heart's effort to maintain the circulation.

A serious high blood pressure, however, is not due to arteriosclerosis. Evidence points to its being caused by uncontrolled and useless contraction of the muscle of the smallest arteries all over the body, thus requiring a much greater effort by the heart to keep the circulation going. The cause is not known. This condition, called "systemic hypertension," remains one of the most important unsolved problems of medicine. It is appearing more and more in people in the younger age groups; it is much more widespread among men than among women.

7. "THE OLD TICKER"

Defects and deterioration in the blood vessels react upon the heart. If the arteries supplying the heart become narrow through "furring" the heart muscle itself cannot get sufficient blood for its own requirements. This expresses itself as an "angina," which merely means "pain." This pain starts over the breast bone and radiates down the inner side of the left arm, sometimes down both arms and into the middle fingers. Every time the person with this condition exerts himself in an effort for which the heart arteries cannot supply sufficient blood, he is sharply reminded by this pain and has to stop. This will happen over and over again until he learns to lead his bodily life in a lower gear. Nature uses this device of pain to pull him up before his heart muscle is dangerously short of oxygen. But there is no scientific explanation why the body should signal in this way any more than there is for the fact that lack of food produces the sensation we call hunger, or lack of water, the sensation we call thirst.

Heart disease is increasing in the highly developed countries at a rate which is alarming; more than a third of all deaths are attributable to the breakdown of this organ. It is the occupational disease of doctors. More doctors die of it than of any other complaint. Obviously it is something to do with the pace of the life we lead and the stresses, fears and alarms of modern existence. In this hot-rod race which we call modern living we are super-charging our engine.

And a very remarkable engine it is, without any super-charging. The heart is very strong and very tough. It has to be if it is to pump blood for a lifetime without stopping for repairs. The toughest metallic machinery could not endure if operated incessantly for seventy years. In the course of that time the heart beats 1,250 million times. Although the average weight of blood in the body is only seven and one half pounds the work done by the heart in twenty-four hours has been calculated at 14,000 kilo-gram-metres—sufficient to raise a 150-pound man to twice the height of the Woolworth Building. It is very willing—in extreme exertion, to meet the body's need for the oxygen carried by the blood, it will treble its output—but apparently it cannot meet our capricious demands. So, however much we may learn about the reasons for heart disease, medicaments will only temporize with the stresses which are sociological and not physiological.

8. STROKE

Failures of the blood supply affect the brain and the nervous system. Once again the wearing-out processes which are understandable in old age are occurring in younger people. One explanation is, with all the benefits of modern medicine and the control of infectious diseases, children with weak constitutions are surviving into adult life and weaknesses may reveal themselves at an age which would be premature in a stronger body. That, however, cannot be the entire explanation and the pace of living must be held responsible for much of the pre-dating of the aging processes.

When an artery is narrowed or hardened it reduces the blood supply to the brain and the part which it supplies will suffer and degenerate. If a clot gets into one of the brain arteries and cuts off the oxygen supply the brain cells will die, and if the victim does not cease to exist entirely the damage to a particular part will produce paralysis. Or the damaged blood vessels may rupture and produce a cerebral hemorrhage. In younger people, at least, these manifestations are due to "systemic hypertension"—that Great Unexplained. Maybe the knowledge of blood-thinners will avoid clotting, and tranquilizers will reduce blood pressure, but these are relieving the condition, without reference to the cause.

9. LOST CONTROL

Sometimes the nervous system wears out prematurely in parts, although its blood supply, as far as can be seen, remains good and the patient is not old by ordinary standards.

A case in point is the failure of the nerve cells at the base of the brain, which exert a strange and still imperfectly understood influence on voluntary movements.

This condition is sometimes known as "shaking paralysis" (*paralysis agitans*) but is medically referred to as *Parkinson's disease,* after James Parkinson, who described it in 1817. It may be due to a number of different disease processes. Occasionally it can follow a head injury; it was a common and permanent complication of sleeping sickness (*encephalitis lethargica*)—a strange disease which has mysteriously died out. It can be due to manganese poisoning. It can occur in later life through the hardening of the arteries which supply the particular nerve cells, but it may start in relatively early adult life because of degeneration of the cells themselves. It reveals itself in stiffness and rigidity of the muscles, causing a delayed action of all voluntary movements, and a tremor, mainly noticeable when the patient is sitting still and disappearing when he is active.

Another mysterious disease of the nervous system is *disseminated sclerosis.* It consists of hardened patches from the size of a pinhead to that of a pea scattered irregularly through the brain and the spinal cord. The insulating sheaths of the nerves are broken down and the nerve cells and fibers have fused together. But why? It is due to the action of some substance which dissolves or breaks up the fatty matter of the nerve sheaths. Having said that, one can only repeat: But why?

Its symptoms usually start with sudden double vision or the temporary paralysis of a limb. Those early symptoms may pass but sooner or later they will recur. The finger wobbles when attempting to touch an object; the hand shakes; the eyes jerk backwards and forwards and the speech is staccato. More and more the patient loses grip and becomes seriously handicapped and bedridden. It is a disease of early adult life, more common among men than women, and is confined to the European races.

Our "unfinished business" includes an unsatisfactory understanding of epilepsy and an imperfect explanation of the ulcers of the stomach and the intestines—trade mark of the twentieth-century successful businessman! It is known what happens but not how or why.

Ulceration of the intestinal tract occurs through the pepsin and hydrochloric acid in normal gastric juice eating into the wall of the stomach and the tubes. Peptic ulcers, therefore, occur in the stomach and the duodenum. In the intestines below that, the gastric acid is rapidly neutralized by the alkaline pancreatic juices. There used to be advertisements which said "There is enough acid in your stomach to burn a hole in a carpet." And on that argument, superficially, it would not be surprising if the acids corroded the stomach. But that is not the nature of the case. You have a stomach which can, by its acids, digest the toughest beefsteak and yet, normally, and through all the hundreds of thousands of years of man's evolution, it does not digest its own delicate lining. To say that the stomach acids suddenly corrode that lining, the mucous membrane, is like saying that sulphuric acid suddenly corroded the glass of its carboy-container. It cannot happen that way. The mucous membrane is chemically non-corrosible. How then does that lining of the stomach or the duodenum become vulnerable to the acids? That is another part of our "unfinished business"; it is not known. Something happens to the internal chemistry of the body and it may well be that mental stresses, producing emotional reactions, cause the glands to inject the chemicals which produce the changes and the ulcers. Once the membrane collapses, then the acids certainly act on the tissues and extend the ulcers, often eating through the tubes with fatal results.

10. ALLERGIES

Our "allergies" are today fit topics for the drawing room or the barroom. People, in their own case, know what allergy is without knowing what it means. By definition it is "a condition of unusual or exaggerated specific susceptibility to a substance which is harmless in similar amounts for the majority of members of the same species." There can be chemical, physical, or mental allergies. A quantity of a drug which would be completely harmless to one person may be fatal to another ("one man's meat is another man's poison"). Some people react more violently to heat or to cold or to sunlight. Mental reactions may be similarly exaggerated—like some people's antipathy to cats, which is more than just a prejudice and produces a real physical reaction—cold sweats or nausea, as in the case of Lord Nelson.

Allergic reactions are varied. Some people are hypersensitive to organic dust and the emanation of animals, especially horses, and suffer from attacks of bronchial spasms when anywhere near them. Others react to the pollens of grasses and suffer from hay fever in the summer. Some are sensitive to the protein in shellfish and, one of the most inconvenient of all, to that in hen's eggs, and get violent gastrointestinal attacks when there is the slightest suspicion of them in their food. Some people are allergic to detergents, to penicillin, to gasoline, or to aspirin, and the symptoms may be different in different people—asthmatic or bronchial spasms, nettle rash, pimples, eczema, catarrh or pains in the joints.

So what? No one can give a categorical explanation of these allergies, although the mechanism of some of them can be explained. The body, as we have seen, tries to repel anything which is foreign to its constitution. All proteins, when they get inside the body without being changed (as they would be by the digestive system), act as *antigens*. In other words they are like germs, which, when they invade the body, cause it to create *antibodies* which will destroy them—that is, if they ever come again after the antibodies have been alerted. If antibody production is rapid and maintained at a higher level, these antigen-antibody reactions take place in the blood, and there are no untoward symptoms. If, on the other hand the production fails or remains consistently low, the antigen diffuses into the cells and the reaction takes place there instead of in the blood. This releases a poisonous substance, *histamine,* and nasty symptoms follow immediately. The reaction is nearly always local (nobody knows why): the bronchi react and produce asthma; the eyes and nose secrete mucus, as in hay fever; and the stomach and the skin react to others.

Allergy can, then, be attributed to the failure of one of the normal defensive mechanisms of the body. But why? Medical science does not know much but since the tendency to particular allergies runs in families, it may be genetic in such cases. But it is also obvious that mental and emotional factors somehow interfere with the chemical production of antibodies. The antibody mechanism is thus being upset by an emotional condition, just as emotional upsets can inhibit the sexual cycle or check the chemical secretions of the stomach.

In many cases doctors can successfully prescribe *antihistamines*, like *mepyramine* and *promethazine,* which cancel out the action of the histamine in the body. Cortisone, from the adrenal cortex, blocks the violent reaction, in the cells, between the antigen and the antibody, and would be prescribed nowadays in a severe attack.

11. STOCKTAKING

Listing "unfinished business" is like a stocktaking in a general store. The novelty lines which attract current attention have "sold well" (medical science is full of cults and vogues) but "old lines" are still on the shelves because they are so familiar we overlook them.

The common cold, for example, is one of the most intractable diseases because it is *common.* And it is common not because it is simple but because it is complex. Some doctors infer a sort of germ-cocktail, a whole mixture of germs, which produce the symptoms of a cold. But call it a "virus cold" instead of a "common cold" and you will get the finances for a research project.

Just as an intelligent tradesman would use market research to find how he would dispose of his "unfinished business," medical science uses statistics. In the assembly of facts and figures, diseases which have been only vague misgivings suddenly become menacing. If general medical statistics show a steep rise, over a number of years, in lung cancer, medical statisticians ask: Why? If they then find that the years of the increase have a correlation with the amount of tobacco consumed, they will probe further. From the study of cases they will find that a large number of men dying of lung cancer have been heavy smokers for a number of years. They will probe still further and find that a greater proportion of lung cancer cases have been addicted to cigarettes than to cigars or pipes. They will incidentally find that lung cancer is less common amongst women, though increasing, and a further correlation will show that women became heavy cigarette smokers more recently than men—and lung cancer is a delayed action. Having found all this, and thoroughly alarmed not only those who smoke cigarettes but those who sell them, they are likely to get large sums of money to investigate the biochemical reasons.

Similarly, if you remind those who dispose of money, either as legislators or as businessmen, that the figures show that tycoons are becoming increasingly more liable to heart disease or duodenal ulcers, there is more likelihood of getting money to "finish the business." This is not intended to be cynical but merely to show that medical statistics are powerful public relations.

Part Twelve

HEALTHY MAN IN A
HEALTHY WORLD

> Any man's *death* diminishes *me*, be-
> cause I am involved in *Mankinde:* And
> therefore never send to know for whom
> the *bell* tolls; It tolls for *thee*.
>
> —JOHN DONNE. *Devotions, XVII*

1. CHEOPIS

A daylight visit to the sculptors' quarter of Calcutta had
the quality of a nightmare. We picked our way through a
jungle of limbs—the arms of Karttikeya, the Hindu God
of War. Booth after booth and stall after stall were devoted to selling and making this extraordinary idol—a
six-headed god riding on a peacock and brandishing a
variety of weapons in his twelve hands.

I said to my companion, a Hindu doctor, that this worship of war seemed to be ominous, but he pointed out
that, on the contrary, it showed a concern for peace. He
reminded me that down at the Kali Ghat, on the River
Hooghli, they offered blood sacrifices and called Kali
"the Gracious Goddess," although she was the symbol
of evil; this was to humor her and distract her from death
and destruction. And so it was with Karttikeya and war-
making; it was a policy of appeasement. This has had its
parallel in medicine—as in Babylon where fiendish images of the gods of disease were set up on the thresholds
of the houses.

Our visit was not concerned with Karttikeya but with
Cheopis, which has, in its time, killed far more people
then war. Cheopis is the flea, the carrier of bubonic
plague—the Black Death, which, according to some estimates, killed half the population of Europe in the fifteenth
century and was responsible for the Great Plague of
London. Through all the centuries it has ravaged the
world.

On the world map of pestilential diseases, Calcutta

figures as one of the few remaining plague centers. The large-scale map does not narrow the focus down, as we were doing, to a comparatively small group of streets in the city. There, behind the sculptors' quarter and the hedge of arms of Karttikeya, bubonic plague slumbers like a sleeping volcano, occasionally throwing up a few cases, sometimes scattering the disease through the city but always liable to erupt like Krakatoa, which when it exploded destroyed an island and scattered its dust across the entire world in 1883. This group of slum streets is one of the few endemic centers which keep the medical officers of the entire world uneasily on the alert.

With us was a Plague Squad and we picked our way through narrow alleys between mud and bamboo huts, adhering like revolting fungi to the walls of warehouses and factories which were themselves slums. We had to clamber over the sick littering the ground; over children squatting and rooting the filth; and over the emaciated cows, lolling in miserable and disease-ridden sanctity. The objective of the Squad was the rats, the breeding-pastures of the fleas. Rats abounded in these slum conditions and they were particularly plentiful in the grain store for which we were heading.

There was no difficulty in finding the ratholes. The members of the Squad sealed as many as they could find, leaving an obvious one into which they pushed a nozzle and injected deadly cyanide gas. Rats came swarming out desperately gasping for air, and died at our feet. Those who were still too lively were clubbed. Some escaped to die elsewhere and an untold many died in the ratholes, which the team filled with bleaching powder. Others of the Squad were quickly covering the corpses with DDT. The cyanide could not kill the fleas, which, escaping from the corpses, might still find human refuges and cause the plague.

Plague can travel as far and as fast as a jet-engined aircraft. Within two days I was back in London. Within three days I could have been in New York. I had been inoculated before I went into the plague spot; I had been dusted with DDT, and, needless to say, I had hurried back to the hotel for a shower and a change of clothes. But it could have happened; I might have picked up a flea, and from it the pestilence; and I might have become a carrier.

2. NO MAN IS AN ISLAND

This story of a rendezvous with Karttikeya and Cheopis in the slums of Calcutta has a moral. No man is self-sufficient. If he has a stomach ulcer, that is just too bad for him; if he has contracted plague from a flea, then it can be bad for many. But even that ulcer may be due to the fact that he is a member of the community; it may derive from his relationship with others—the stress of the ticker tape or the telephone, or the emotional upset of a board meeting or a family row.

As John Donne said "no man is an island." So far, this book has tried to show how man acquired the knowledge of the fabric of his body—the skeleton, the muscles, the organs, the nerves, the brain and the glands, and it ought to have shown that the Whole Man is something more than a kit containing a collection of separate items. His mind and his body, his glands and his brain, his nerves and his blood vessels, and his health and his temperament are all interrelated. What he is and how he feels depends on the interplay of all of them. But his internal economy depends on external relations.

He is the product of his ancestry—which goes back to the amoeba ingesting its sustenance from the primeval slime. He is a product of the air he breathes, of the sun that warms him, of the water he drinks, of the food he eats, and of the soil in which that food grows. He lives in competition, and in constant war, with the inhabitants of the Rival World—micro-organisms, the insects and the pests—and when his defenses break, he, the individual, can lose the battle to such enemies, which bring disease and hunger.

Man has never been independent of the group. The family is as real a biological unit as he is himself. The family expands into the tribe—not just a collection of individuals, like a crowd at a ball game, but biologically involved. (This is recognized in primitive tribes, with their totems and taboos to guard against incest, with its risks of inheritance of bad characteristics.) When the tribes settle as city-cultures, the medical hazards increase.

Wandering tribes do not have to worry about sanitary disposal of waste. Water drunk from a spring or running stream is unlikely to have water-borne infection. There

233

are risks even among the nomads but less of man-to-man infection or contagion. Until the white man took his community infections into the Arctic contagious disease was rare, if not entirely absent, among the Eskimos—to the extent that they had no immunity whatever, so that a common cold could be as lethal as cholera. Their tribulations were hunger and the diseases they contracted from the food they ate—hydatid diseases through eating the parasites in uncooked meat; tularemia, the rodent disease, contracted from the Arctic hare, and brucellosis, which causes abortion in animals and undulant fever in man.

With the growth of settled communities, however, communicable diseases became a menace. Sewage infections; defiled water; insect-borne diseases, carrying parasites from one diseased person to another; flies, picking up human diseases and contaminating human food; fleas and lice, loaded with disease, and brushed off the rags of the beggar onto the robes of a passing prince; contact diseases like leprosy and syphilis; and air-borne diseases, like the sneeze which passes on influenza—all these came with the crowding and congestion of people into towns.

The ancient civilizations had an awareness of these. That is obvious from the Book of Leviticus in the Bible; from Nergal, the Babylonian Fly God; the Minoan sewage pits; the ruthless segregation of lepers, and the great fresh-water aqueducts of Rome. They had an awareness which was forgotten in the Middle Ages.

3. THE GREAT SANITARY AWAKENING

The modern public health movement was foreshadowed by Johann Peter Frank (1745-1821). This German, a poor waif abandoned on a doorstep, made himself one of the great public health teachers of all times. His work on public hygiene covered the whole subject of man's life "from the womb to the tomb"—sewerage, water supply, school hygiene, and even the taxation of bachelors, as well as a concept of medical police—the medical officer of health.

But the Great Sanitary Awakening began about 1850 with the epoch-making report by Sir Edwin Chadwick on

The Sanitary Condition of the Labouring Population of Great Britain. He recognized that a country, however superficially prosperous, could not continue to exist half-rich and half-poor, half-sick and half-well. It was clear to him and the other early pioneers that poverty and disease form a vicious circle. Men and women were sick because they were poor; they became poorer because they were sick and sicker because they were poorer. A century ago it came to be recognized that the wealth of a nation was the health of its people and that the pursuit of happiness was the pursuit of well-being.

With the realization that wealth could not buy immunity from diseases bred in poverty came the recognition that preventive medicine was a charge upon the community, which had to make itself responsible for services which were a common risk or a common benefit for all. This meant public sewage and water systems; sanitary codes for housing; factory legislation to reduce not only industrial hazards but conditions of work liable to breed disease; quarantine measures to help to close ports to imported diseases; and the development of isolation hospitals and sanatoria to remove active cases of contagion and infection which might spread through the community.

Out of *preventive* health measures came the idea of *positive* health. This meant not only the better planning of towns and the proper provision of open spaces, but the application of nutrition—ensuring that at least the growing generations would have a well-nourished body to resist disease. This meant school feeding and supplementary diets for children and adolescents.

The British have carried the logic of Chadwick even further in the National Health Service, which includes not only *preventive* and *positive* medicine, through public health and social services, but a *sickness* service as well. From before birth until death, the individual can have a complete medical service and medical attention as a taxpayer's right. The service comprehends everything, from prenatal clinics to geriatric hospitals for old people and the services of the general practitioners and the consultants and the facilities of the hospital services.

4. THE COST OF SICKNESS

With the recognition that Health is Wealth, enlightened countries began to look at their health balance sheets.

The values of human health are not to be measured in financial terms alone. As the preamble to the constitution of the World Health Organization states, the enjoyment of the highest attainable standard of health is one of the fundamental rights of every human being. And it is manifestly true that those burdened with ill health cannot find a full expression of their personality or make a full contribution to their community.

The first measure of the economic burden of disease in a given country is the mean life expectancy of its population. How premature death can be controlled is shown by the experience in those countries which have a public health program of long standing. The oldest mortality records available are those of Sweden. In that country the expectation of life in 1755-76 was thirty-four years. With improved conditions it had risen to forty-one years by 1840. But with the rapid development of public health science in the nineteenth century it had risen to fifty-seven years in 1920 and sixty-six years in 1940. The expectation of human life had been doubled. In the U.S.A., the mean life expectancy at the beginning of this century was forty-eight years for males and fifty-one years for females. At the mid-century the corresponding figures were sixty-five and seventy-one respectively.

What is the money value of a man? It has been estimated (Dublin, Lotka and Spiegelman, 1947) that, taking into account the drain upon family and community, Junior represents a considerable financial investment, in anticipation of a productive return in later life. For a family with a $2,500 annual income, it costs $10,000 to maintain and educate a child to the age of eighteen. It has been shown that, for the high-income groups in the U.S.A., the peak of earning capacity is not reached till the age of fifty-five; and, for low-income groups, it is reached at thirty-five to forty. For those low-income groups, which represent the greater part of the American population, the curve of earnings does not vary much be-ween twenty-five and sixty-five. Thus, a death at fifteen ears of age represents a net economic loss to society; a eath at forty represents a net economic gain, but a death t sixty-five represents a net gain more than twice as reat.

In countries such as China, Egypt and India, where he average expectation of life is in the neighborhood f thirty years, only fifty-four out of every one hundred hildren born ever reach the age of fifteen and enter on he period of maximum productivity.

Apart from premature death, sickness and disease are drain on the prosperity even of the wealthiest coun- ries. The U.S. Public Health Service, in a national health urvey, showed that on any given day 4.5 per cent of the American population were so disabled by illness or physi- al or emotional handicap as to be unable to go to work. One per cent of the entire population had been incapaci- ated for a full year at the time of the survey.

In 1949, when the U.S.A. had a total national income f $217,000,000,000, five per cent of it, $10,600,000,- 00, was spent on the medical and institutional care of he diseased. Paresis, nervous disorders involving com- lete or partial paralysis, means, in the United States, he staggering loss of income of $112,000,000 a year. And the estimated cost of temporary or permanent dis- bility from all causes is between $3,000,000,000 and 4,000,000,000 annually in the U.S.A.

If we cynically to disregard the suffering and misery which those figures conceal, we might say that a wealthy country like the United States can afford to pay per cent of its national income on the care of the sick not the prevention of ill-health) and on the loss of pro- ductivity, but that is certainly not true of less prosperous ountries. Certainly poor Ecuador cannot afford the $30,- 00,000—12.5 per cent of its national income—lost very year through premature death, disablement and emporary incapacity through illness. Egypt (national in- ome, $1,800,000,000) cannot afford to lose a third of ts productive capacity and $60,000,000 a year through ne disease, bilharziasis. Nor India (national income, 17,000,000,000) the $240,000,000 which malaria costs nnually; nor the Philippines (national income, $2,334,- 00,000) the $660,000,000 lost annually through ma- aria and tuberculosis.

5. STUB THAT BUTT!

Every year, millions of acres of standing timber are destroyed by forest fires in Canada and the United States.

In North Saskatchewan, I was watching the Smoke Jumpers practicing their parachute leaps, which would take them and their fire-fighting equipment out of the aircraft and into the heart of the forest. And I asked Earl Dodds, the Field Officer who was with me, "Is this the most efficient way of fighting forest fires?"

"No," said Earl, "the most efficient way is to stub the cigarette butt before it starts the forest fire."

That is a sound slogan for health services as well: "Stub that butt!"

Prevention is infinitely cheaper than *cure*. But *positive* health is a better investment than either. If, with healthy housing, sound nutrition, and opportunities for fresh air and exercise, you avoid—from the start—the social conditions which promote the disease, you do not have the costly business of prevention, treatment and eradication.

What is more, as the best employers now know, good food and good conditions, apart from reducing the costs of medical services, are a good investment in themselves. In the High Arctic, where military construction work was going on, the cost of feeding the construction men, I found, was $15 a day, allowing not only for the cost of flying in the T-bone steaks and fresh vegetables, but the fuel oil and the dieticians. I remarked to one superintendent that this sounded very costly. His reply was:

"And so is stainless steel, but it is cheaper in the long run than putting in steel that will rust and undo your work."

With modern knowledge of nutritional science, that should be obvious, but the general attitude is still like that of his medical contemporaries denouncing Oliver Wendell Holmes for daring to suggest that they should clean their hands before delivering a baby.

When, no longer ago than 1947, an Expert Committee of the Food and Agriculture Organization suggested that proper food for the workers on development schemes being internationally assisted, should be costed as part of

he capital investment of, say, a dam, the idea was
ttacked as revolutionary and "unsound finance."

This attitude has been modified in terms of "social
ngineering" in the schemes for technical assistance and
nutual aid and what President Truman described as "A
3old New Program" for making science and technology
vailable to the underdeveloped countries. The criterion
•f such aid is basically that any assistance should pro-
luce economic returns, but that is now accepted as in-
luding better food, better health measures, and better
ducational facilities.

While remembering that the sensible thing is to "stub
•ut the butt," we still need the medical "fire-watchers"
—like that Plague Squad killing off the rats and the
leas in Calcutta (although it would be better still to pull
lown the slums in which they breed).

Every town and city, in any country which professes
o be enlightened, now recognizes the need for those
·igilantes, the public health men, the food inspectors and
he sanitarians. Every country, even many which are re-
;arded as backward, has measures of national protec-
ion—port and air-terminal and frontier medical officers,
o see that suspect carriers do not get through; quaran-
ine ordinances to isolate any who may have contracted
•n infectious or contagious disease; and organization for
lealing with an outbreak if it occurs.

Such measures are desperately necessary. A single case
•f a pestilential disease may wreak havoc even within a
vell-organized country. When a passenger arriving at an
•irport is asked to give in detail where he has been, where
•e has spent the past four nights, and precisely where he
s going, it is not officious inquisitiveness. If a case of dis-
:ase should be reported from where he has been, if he
.hould himself develop symptoms, or if someone in the
ocality to which he is going should later develop them
(even if the passenger does not) the medical authorities
vill be swift to act—and the swifter the better. The pas-
•enger may be a "carrier," one who infects others with a
lisease without suffering from it.

6. TYPHOID MARY

The most famous, or notorious, "carrier" was "Typhoid Mary."

In 1901 Mary Mallon, a cook, was employed by a family in New York City. A visitor to the home fell ill with typhoid. A month later, the family laundress also came down with it.

In 1902 Mary Mallon moved to another place, and two weeks after her arrival a fellow-servant had typhoid; then another, and then all seven members of the family.

In 1904 the cook went to a household in Long Island. Within three weeks of her arrival, four of the servants had the fever.

In 1906 she took service with another family and six of the eleven members were infected. Here she was first suspected of being a carrier and left. Three weeks later, in her new place, another laundress was taken ill.

In 1907 she was back again in New York and again typhoid occurred in the household.

During those five years, "Typhoid Mary" is known to have been the cause of twenty-five cases of typhoid fever, and it is believed that she may have been responsible for the New York outbreak of 1903 when there were 1,300 victims.

She was put into hospital under supervision by the New York City Department of Health but broke her promise to report regularly and give up her profession of cook. Soon, twenty-five cases of typhoid broke out among the staff of the Sloane Hospital, New York. The cook left in a hurry without disclosing her address. The hunt began and at last she was found, living, like a fugitive criminal, under an assumed name. She was given a good job in the Department of Health Laboratories, where they could keep an eye on her, and remained there until she died, twenty years later.

7. INSECT HOBOES

Another danger is the speed of modern travel—insects can stow away and take their disease-baggage with them.

In 1930, some mosquito-hoboes hitched a ride on an aircraft from West Africa to Brazil—a distance of 2,000 miles. They carried malaria and caused an epidemic of 300,000 cases, of whom 16,000 died. Since then, the Brazilian authorities have been rigid in their regulations. All aircraft are thoroughly examined. Passengers may find it exasperating to sit stewing in an aircraft on the blistering tarmac, in a cabin with all the airholes sealed, while sanitarians search for mosquitoes like customs officers looking for contraband, and they may resent the exploding of fumigation bombs which make them cough and splutter. But such discomfort is a minor concern compared with the risks and with the fact that in three years 68,000 insects, including 352 malaria-carriers, were found on aircraft from Africa. If one of those anopheles had escaped death at the airport, the deadly epidemic might have been repeated.

8. CALLING ALL GERMS

At the center of the global defense strategy against pestilence is the World Health Organization's epidemiological service.

As soon as it was set up as one of the U.N. agencies after the war, WHO set about organizing the fastest possible system of reporting the movements of disease, particularly of the old "killers," the pestilential diseases, plague, cholera, smallpox, yellow fever and typhus.

From almost any part of the world, it will learn of an outbreak within a few hours. This information is relayed from special wireless stations at Singapore, Washington and Alexandria. The control office at the Palais des Nations in Geneva receives these messages and beams a daily bulletin all over the world from Prangins Radio Station. The main network of radio stations is supported by numerous relay stations which pick up and retransmit the information. All messages are sent in code—to prevent eavesdroppers from spreading alarm and despondency—and, now, in addition to the alerting on the pestilentials, the daily bulletins include information about any of 135 diseases.

That is a general warning service, but in addition special warnings are telegraphed to any countries likely to be exposed to special risk. How necessary this is, is instanced by the case of Singapore, which is at the eastern crossroads of shipping and air traffic. Through it, craft pass to

360 ports and airports and the general warning may not be fast enough or specific enough when a ship or an aircraft is found to have a suspected case on board. In that event the ship itself would be warned "on information received" and its next port of call warned "prepare for quarantine."

This service is not purely negative—not just a matter of warning port authorities to apply restrictions; it is also valuable in calling off restrictions without unnecessary delays, which annoy travelers and hold up trade.

The World Health Organization is the Department of Health for the whole world. It has no powers and no sanctions and can work only through governments, but its authority is vested in the inescapable truth that *disease knows no frontiers*. In this, at least, nations must work together.

To its valuable functions of collecting and disseminating facts and medical knowledge; preparing pharmacopeia, so that a patient moving round the world can be sure that his regimen can be maintained wherever he is; standardizing drugs; investigating diseases, like influenza; bringing experts together to teach each other and promote advances, WHO has a tactical role as well. Mankind cannot properly measure the ineffable benefits which WHO, often in close conjunction with the United Nations Children's Fund, has conferred in the few years of its existence —cannot measure, because its greatest achievements are expressed not in what has happened but *what did not happen*.

By disposing its experts and dispensing the wonders of modern drugs, it has cured millions, directly protected millions, and indirectly protected hundreds of millions.

9. *COUNTERATTACK*

The attack on the massive disease problems which have burdened and crippled nations is direct—like insecticides to get rid of malaria, antibiotics to deal with syphilis or yaws, or B.C.G. to protect those exposed to tuberculosis.

Massive—and expensive. But nothing like the expense of disease. Before the war, Greece used to spend $1,300,-000 a year on quinine to reduce the effects of malaria;

today malaria has been banished and is kept out of Greece at a cost of $300,000 for DDT. Leaving out of account the loss of productivity and earnings, now redressed, the direct saving is a million dollars annually. Haiti, with international help, launched a campaign against yaws, with the result that 100,000 incapacitated people were able to work again, adding $5,000,000 to the *annual* income. The *total* cost of the campaign was $800,000. In Venezuela, the intervention of two WHO sanitary experts to provide safe water meant, apart from the relief from the miseries of water-borne diseases, a measurable financial profit of 800 per cent annually. And so and so on . . .

The saying that the health of a people is the wealth of a people is not a pious aphorism. Certainly the converse is true—that a community burdened by ill-health is an impoverished country. There is that vicious circle: disease —underproduction—poverty—poor health services—more disease. That circle is manifest in those underdeveloped countries where the majority of people are afflicted with gross diseases which rob them of vitality and initiative and which create social lethargy. A peasant, sick of a fever at the critical periods of planting and harvesting, cannot grow enough food, or earn enough to buy it. Malnutrition in turn exposes him to infectious and other diseases, and not only are he and his family impoverished but all the standards of his community are degraded physically and in morale. The control of disease is the first step to positive health, which is defined in the Universal Declaration of Human Rights as: "Everyone has the right to a standard of living adequate for the health and well-being of himself and his family, including food, clothing, housing and medical care." That is the precondition of economic and social development. The advance of any community depends on the extent to which it reduces the burden of ill health, which squanders human resources, wastes food in nourishing bacteria and parasites, produces social apathy and prevents people, and nations, from developing their full capacities.

When I undertook a mission to Southeast Asia, descriptively called *Men Against Disease,* my original terms of reference would have confined me to the disease-fighting activities of WHO, which was sending me. The then Director General, Dr. Brock Chisholm, demurred. He said that combating disease was not the concern only of the medical agency of the United Nations; it involved food (FAO) and ignorance (UNESCO) and conditions of work (ILO) and all the social endeavors of the United Nations. And so I went for all of them.

10. "COMPLETE WELL-BEING"

So we have in the World Health Organization a body committed, perforce, by a world full of sickness, to the combating of disease, but dedicated to a greater fulfillment, which is expressed in terms of its own charter, which defines health as: "A state of complete physical, mental and social well-being, and not merely the absence of disease or infirmities."

Notice particularly the word "mental." The world could be rid entirely of disease and physical infirmity and people would still not be happy. Sweden has one of the finest health services in the world and its suicide rate is among the highest. In the United States and Britain the rise of mental illness and the neuroses is alarming.

It is not just the trappings of social well-being that we need but the realities. The hectic pace of modern living and all the gadgetry which goes with it and the urgent discontent of new-found and unsatisfied desires are taking their toll.

Once, with a philosopher friend, I was driving along an American parkway on a Sunday. We were jogging along but on the adjoining fast lane, glittering, high-powered cars were streaking past us and my friend said: "See all those people? They are running away from themselves and don't realize that they are taking themselves with them."

There is the rub. Medical science can give us absence of sickness but it cannot give us health. The resources of our own industry and our own community can give us all the physical components—better sanitation, efficient medical services, better housing, better towns, but it has been said: "Others can provide a house for you but they can never make it a home." Similarly, health in the last analysis depends not on services but on self.

Man is the creature of his environment, and his individuality depends on coming to terms with it. That is a tough proposition in the world today, when events which beset the ordinary man are so often determined by men who, whatever their capacities or eminence, are still flesh and blood, nerves and glands and bodies which react on minds, and minds that react on bodies.

11. HISTORY IS A CLINICAL TEXTBOOK

Between the two World Wars, Professor Sir David Wilkie, a famous surgeon, said to me:

"Whole chapters of history might have been changed by the doctor or surgeon. If attached to the Treaty of Versailles we could have had a clinical history of the signatories we might find an extremely simple and illuminating explanation of its faults. The caution which we applaud as wisdom in elder statesmen, we would often find is due to physical causes, and very often it is enlargement of the prostate, and disorder of the kidney function. We demand physical fitness of the men we send to fight but we make no such demand in regard to those who commit them to battle, or of those whose policies and capacities for quick decision and prompt action control the destinies of nations and the lives of men."

That is not a wayward thought. Statesmen and men of affairs today are shockingly overworked. Momentous decisions depend upon the few and no armies of officials or assistants can temper the psychosomatic effects of the strains of decisions upon the body or the pains of the body upon decisions. A mortally ill Chamberlain went to Munich; a dying Roosevelt went to Yalta; chancelleries rocked and policies tottered when Eisenhower had a heart attack, and diplomatic bags later carried the most intimate clinical details of his ileac disease; a sick and suffering Eden took the decision on Suez, and Foster Dulles, hospitalized with a serious surgical operation, had to decide on a policy for the Middle East.

12. MAN'S LAST ENEMY

There is abounding promise in medical knowledge, but knowledge is not wisdom—wisdom is knowledge tempered by judgment. We can use all the medical knowledge and the more that is to come to get rid of all the natural enemies which produce disease and infirmity and find that man's last enemy is man himself.

Man's challenge, above all others, is the use he makes of the nuclear energy which his ingenuity has released, like the genie from the bottle, to serve him or destroy him. The risks of atomic energy are medical as well as military. A nuclear war would be the suicide pact of the human race, but the hazards are not confined to war.

Without arguing the pros and cons of H-bomb tests, they have at least served to inform the world at large of the facts of radiation and of radioactive dust permeating the atmosphere, which is common to everyone on the planet. There is an awareness that in addition to *somatic* effects, harmful to the individual exposed to them, there are *genetic* effects, which may affect future generations.

Thus man, while solving his medical problems, is himself creating new ones. The atom holds out its benevolent promise of power for prosperity and with its isotopes to explain the inner mysteries of the living body and to treat its weaknesses. The release of its energy has initiated what Professor W. E. Mayneord, of the Royal Marsden Hospital, London, described at the U.N. Atoms-for-Peace Conference as "Humanity's greatest adventure."

But, as he added, all adventure has an element of risk.

The biologists are aware of those risks. Their knowledge of the genetic hazards of nuclear radiations is still imperfect and that is all the more reason why the margins of safety should be large, even to the degree of exaggerated caution.

Industrial atomic energy plants will multiply, as they should. They will spread out all over the world—as they should, for atomic energy is needed in power-hungry, underdeveloped countries. They will, as the intensive British power-station program already demands, be sited near population centers. They will increasingly produce radioactive wastes, which, though not a serious disposal problem today, may become so as the numbers of stations increase. Those wastes are themselves useful and valuable and could have a world-wide use as radioactive isotopes, but to disperse them in that way is only to dispose of them more widely, and that demands safeguards and competence in those who use them.

All these are public health problems of a new order, and since radiation, like disease, knows no frontiers they cannot be settled in a locality or a country or a continent, but only by international conventions in which the levels are defined and enforced and through which supervision can be exercised. There will have to be international agreements on the conditions of work in atomic factories and atomic power plants. There will have to be new education of the local medical officers of the Atomic Age and nuclear health instruction for the ordinary people—if for no other reason than to reassure them that everything is "under control."

These are things which industrialists cannot be allowed to decide for themselves; nor national governments. In the Commonwealth of the Atom there must be collective health security, through the international agencies of the United Nations.

Such decisions, involving not only ourselves but posterity, require the knowledge, the judgment, and the wisdom of mature men and women. Dr. Brock Chisholm, when he was Director General of the World Health Organization, defined a mature person as "one who can think two generations ahead." Such people are in short supply in an age in which we are all preoccupied with this morning's headlines, next week's pay envelope, or how we can afford to put Junior through college. We have not got around to thinking of paying installments on posterity.

Descartes said: "If there is any possible means of increasing the common wisdom and ability of mankind, it must be sought in medicine." Indeed it must, for it is the Science of Humanity.

INDEX